Young Black Women and Health Inequities in the United States

This important book not only highlights the high rates of morbidity and mortality among young Black women in the United States but also provides a lens through which the reasons behind such health disparities can be understood.

The book outlines the main direct causes of illness and premature death among young Black women, from physical illnesses such as heart disease, cancer, and stroke, to psychological conditions such as depression. But throughout each chapter, the reasons behind these issues are discussed, including exposure to racial discrimination, exposure to psychosocial stressors, poverty, lack of access to health care, unemployment, and lack of education. A concluding chapter asks what mechanisms can address the stark health inequities faced by young Black women in the United States so that rates of morbidity and mortality can be reduced.

A timely and insightful account of an enduring issue within American society, this book will interest researchers and students across public health, race, and gender studies and the sociology of health, as well as policy makers and policy-makers.

Suezanne Tangerose Orr, M.A., Ph.D., received her Ph.D. in Epidemiology from the University of North Carolina (Chapel Hill). She has been a faculty member at the University of Maryland School of Medicine, the Johns Hopkins University School of Public Health, and the East Carolina University College of Health and Human Performance and School of Medicine. At each of these Universities, she taught graduate courses focused upon Psychosocial and Behavioral Aspects of Health; Race, Ethnicity, and Disease; Research Methods; and Introduction to Epidemiology.

Caroline Orr Bueno, M.A., M.S., Ph.D., completed her Ph.D. in Social and Behavioral Sciences at Virginia Commonwealth University in December 2020. She is currently a Postdoctoral Fellow at the University of Maryland, College Park. She also holds an M.A. degree in Health Education and Promotion from East Carolina University and an M.S. degree in Counseling Psychology from Loyola University (Baltimore).

Young Black Women and Health Inequities in the United States

A Social Determinants Approach

Suezanne Tangerose Orr and Caroline Orr Bueno

Routledge
Taylor & Francis Group
LONDON AND NEW YORK

Designed cover image: Routledge

First published 2024
by Routledge
4 Park Square, Milton Park, Abingdon, Oxon OX14 4RN

and by Routledge
605 Third Avenue, New York, NY 10158

Routledge is an imprint of the Taylor & Francis Group, an informa business

British Library Cataloguing-in-Publication Data
A catalogue record for this book is available from the British Library

Library of Congress Cataloging-in-Publication Data
A catalog record for this book has been requested

ISBN: 978-1-032-26780-7 (hbk)
ISBN: 978-1-032-66379-1 (pbk)
ISBN: 978-1-032-66380-7 (ebk)

DOI: 10.4324/9781032663807

Typeset in Sabon
by Apex CoVantage, LLC

Dedication

I was encouraged and inspired to write this book due to the many blessings in my life of family, colleagues, mentors, and friends. The book is dedicated, with love, to these people, who have played such an important role in my life and work.

My parents, James and Elizabeth Tangerose, provided me with a foundation of love, self-confidence, and encouragement. They fostered a love of learning and gave me the gift of a wonderful education. They also created awareness of those who are less fortunate and our obligation to make the world a better place.

My two children, Jamie and Caroline, add so much joy and love to my life. They were wonderful children and are wonderful adults. I am very proud of them, and the caring people they have become. They gave me the gift of five loving grandchildren, who fill my heart with joy. Evangeline, my beautiful granddaughter, sends me to bed every night with a smile on my face after she blows kisses to me and tells me she loves me. I want to make the world a better place for my wonderful children and grandchildren to live.

My wonderful mentor, Professor, colleague, collaborator, and friend of over 40 years, Sherman James, Ph.D., has always, despite his very busy life as a brilliant Social Epidemiologist, generously made time to help, support, advise, and encourage me. He was my Advisor in graduate school, Chair of my doctoral Dissertation Committee, and is a treasured mentor, friend, and colleague. My life and work are better from the gift of knowing and collaborating with Sherman and having him as a friend.

The late C. Arden Miller, M.D., also was a wonderful mentor, colleague, collaborator, Professor, and friend. He was a great source of information, ideas, support, help, and encouragement. He inspired me very early in my career to focus my interest in research about racial disparities in health and the relationship between psychosocial factors with health on issues related to pregnancy. It was a great honor to have Arden as a friend and collaborator.

To these individuals, and many others I was blessed to have as friends and colleagues (especially Drs. David Kleinbaum and Dan Blazer), I thank you for your love, kindness, guidance, friendship, and contributions to my life and work.

Suezanne T. Orr, M.A., Ph.D.

Dedication

To my mom, Dr. Suezanne Orr, whose lifelong commitment to racial and social justice lit a spark of passion in me as a child that continues to inspire me to this day. To follow in her footsteps is one of the greatest honors of my life.

To the activists and educators who taught me what it means to "show up and do the work" – and then to do it again the next day, for this work never ends. It's an honor and a privilege to learn from you.

To the readers of this book. May this work inspire you to become the next generation of changemakers working to create a healthier, more just society.

Caroline Orr Bueno, M.A., M.S., Ph.D.

Contents

Foreword

Dr. Suezanne T. Orr and Dr. Caroline Orr Bueno have approached racial inequities and the social determinants of health in an enlightened epidemiologic manner. It is not the biological differences between the races that need to be examined. Race is not merely a risk factor for poor health. Rather, including race as a variable in scientific research allows one to examine the components of health that are impacted by the circumstances of racial differences in life's experiences. That is to say, race is a risk *marker* for investigating and considering alternative explanations for the health experiences of young Black women.

This book is a magnificent compilation of decades of research about a multitude of instances in which health disparities between young Black women and young White women exist. It covers exposures to stressors, the phenomena of "weathering," economic instability, pregnancy outcomes along with infant mortality and maternal health, cardiovascular and cerebrovascular differences, malignant neoplasms, depression, sexually transmitted diseases, homicide, health care, and the COVID-19 pandemic.

The authors conclude that the late Dr. Arden Miller and Dr. Jessie Bierman were ahead of their time in recognizing half a century ago the need for societal changes to improve the health of the nation. I would propose that these remarkable scientists were actually right on time for advocating that public health pay attention to the *social determinants of health* that have more recently become "buzz words" to explain the effects of decades of institutional racism. We must be willing to discuss racism as an institutional norm in order to effectively combat its effects on the health of Black women. What is racism? Own it! Not until this nation has the political will to stop denying the existence of social, environmental, and legal policies that shape the health of Black women can meaningful improvements be made. This timely book prioritizing the needs of young Black women is on the right path to elucidate the factors that must be addressed to resolve the myriad of health inequalities faced by young Black women in the United States. Finally, true champions for understanding and improving the health of Black women has arrived.

CAPT Cheryl Blackmore Prince, PhD, MPH, MS
USPHS (Retired)

Dr. Cheryl Blackmore Prince began her decades-long career at the Centers for Disease Control and Prevention (CDC) by completing the two-year Epidemic Intelligence Service (EIS) program. After her service in the EIS, she began her work at the CDC as an epidemiologist, primarily in the Division of Reproductive Health.

She received her doctoral degree in Epidemiology from the School of Public Health at the University of North Carolina, Chapel Hill, in 1992, and her MPH from Emory University in 1987.

At CDC, she was involved with several major scientific programs, such as the Pregnancy Risk Assessment Monitoring System. She was also assigned to Hawaii for a decade to address problems with maternal health and pregnancy.

She has numerous publications in highly regarded peer-reviewed journals and was also part of The Society for the Analysis of African-American Public Health Issues. Her work has focused upon the health and pregnancies of young Black women for decades and is highly respected by scholars in Epidemiology, Public Health, and Obstetrics and Gynecology.

1 Introduction

Young Black Women

Young Black women (ages 15–44 years) play very important roles in their families and communities in the United States. They are mothers, wives, sisters, friends who support other women, caregivers for older parents or grandparents, pillars of their churches, economic wage earners, and essential workers in jobs that provide important services to the community (e.g., teachers, food industry workers, bus drivers, day care workers, nurses and other staff in health care settings, volunteers at their churches and neighborhood schools). Despite the significant roles played by Black women in their families and communities, they were described in a speech by the late civil rights activist Malcolm X in 1962 as "neglected" and "disrespected" (1).

"Essential workers" are those who work in industries that are considered essential for the survival of society, including health care (2). Despite being about 12 percent of the population in the United States, Blacks comprise over one-third of nursing assistants (primarily Black women) (3). Sadly, as one author notes, Black women are "essential but undervalued" (3, 4).

Health of Young Black Women

As the pandemic of COVID-19 swept across the United States beginning in 2020, Black women were far more likely than White women to be hospitalized or to die from this infection (5–10). The only group more likely to be hospitalized or to die from COVID-19 than Black women was Black men (6, 7). The recognition of the disproportionate burden of severe illness or death from COVID-19 among Black compared to White women shone a light on long-standing inequities in health between Black and White women (11–17) and created an awakening to injustice and inequities in health in the United States. Long-standing racism and health inequities in the United States created the circumstances of a pandemic, which disproportionately affected Blacks, and widespread unemployment created by the pandemic also disproportionately affected Blacks (11). It was clear that the same groups who bore a disproportionate burden of severe illness or death from COVID-19,

DOI:10.4324/9781032663807-1

such as Black women, suffered a disproportionate burden from many other health conditions (11, 12, 17–19). The presence of underlying health problems, such as hypertension or diabetes, increased the risk of severe disease or death from COVID-19. Black women have an increased risk of many such chronic health conditions compared to White women (20).

There have been significant (and increasing) disparities in health between Black and White women in the United States for decades (11, 12, 15, 16). However, the pandemic of COVID-19 called increased attention to these disparities (11). As cases of COVID-19 spread and caused death, severe illness, and hospitalizations, Blacks in the United States were more likely than Whites to become hospitalized or to die (5, 6).

Health "disparities" refers to differences in health (morbidity and mortality) between groups. The March of Dimes defines "health disparities" as a circumstance in which health outcomes differ between groups (21). For example, one group might have higher mortality from COVID-19 than another. One of the major objectives of Healthy People 2010 was to reduce health disparities between Blacks and Whites during the next decade (22).

Williams and Purdie-Vaughns called reducing racial disparities in health one of the major public health challenges of our time (23). The Robert Wood Johnson Foundation recently stated that the public health community has an important role to play in the future to dismantle structural barriers to health equity, including structural racism (see later) (24). These significant activities will help all US citizens to achieve their best possible health. The Centers for Disease Control and Prevention (CDC) has also undertaken activities and programs to address health equity.

Health "inequities" refer to circumstances in which members of a group, such as Black women, are unfairly and unjustly denied the opportunity to achieve their best possible health. Inequities in health are disparities that are avoidable, preventable, and unjust. For example, poverty or racial discrimination may unjustly prevent individuals from achieving their best possible health. In the case of COVID-19, there are clear disparities between Black and White women in severe illness and death (5, 6). These inequities are overwhelmingly caused by social, economic, and other unjust circumstances that prevent Black women from achieving optimal health (23).

Social Determinants of Health

In the early 1900s, many deaths in the United States were caused by infectious diseases, such as tuberculosis, influenza, pneumonia, and cholera. Life expectancy at birth in 1900 for White women was 48.7 years, and for Black women, life expectancy at birth was 33.5 years, a difference of over 15 years. It was recognized that social, economic, work, and living conditions played a major role in the spread of infectious diseases in the United States (15, 17, 25, 26). The demographic shift that occurred at this time, of people moving from rural areas (especially in the South) to cities in the Northeast and Midwest in search of jobs as the economy became increasingly industrialized and less agrarian, led to widespread poverty, crowded living conditions, lack of sanitation, and hazardous working conditions in urban areas. For Blacks, these noxious conditions in social and physical environments were magnified by racial discrimination, which created segregated neighborhoods with concentrated poverty, crowded living conditions, poor sanitation, and disease (27).

During the first half of the twentieth century, scientific advances, including the discovery of antibiotics to treat bacterial infections, and the development of public health (e.g., improved hygiene and sanitation), led to great improvement in population health, as demonstrated by increases in life expectancy at birth. However, despite improvements in life expectancy at birth, there remained large disparities in health between Black and White women (11, 26). In 2000, the difference in life expectancy at birth between Black and White women in the United States was close to five years (see Chapter 2). A report by the National Research Council described health of Americans compared to citizens of other wealthy nations as "Shorter Lives, Poorer Health" (28). A primary reason for the poorer health (see Chapter 2) of Americans is the detrimental impact of the social, environmental, cultural, and political environment in the United States, especially for Blacks (28, 29).

It was believed by some that continued scientific and technological advances in medicine and public health would continue to bring about improvements in the health of the American population (12, 16). However, the same social conditions that allowed infectious diseases to spread in the early 1900s (e.g., poverty, overcrowded housing) continued to negatively impact the health of Americans, especially Blacks (9, 12, 26, 28, 29). It is estimated that only 10 to 20 percent of health outcomes can be attributed to health care factors (26, 30, 31) and that changes in social, political, educational, and economic policies would bring about far more improvements in the health of Americans than increased investment in health care (30).

In recent decades, researchers in fields such as Public Health, Social Epidemiology, and Sociology noted the disparities in indicators of health between Blacks and Whites in the United States. As a result of this work, in 1985, the Secretary of the Department of Health and Human Services (DHHS), Margaret Heckler, released a report on Black and Minority Health, known as the Heckler Report (32). This report identified large health disparities between Whites and members of groups of other races/ethnicities (32). Following this report, in 1986, the United States Department of Health and Human Services established the Office of Minority Health.

Research showed that individual risk factors or behaviors could not explain racial disparities in health. Additionally, health care only accounts for a small part of population health and health disparities (28, 31). In order to understand and reduce health disparities between Blacks and Whites, it is necessary to focus upon social factors that have widespread impacts upon health and health outcomes, such as systemic racism, poverty, and exposure to chronic stressful life conditions (23, 26, 29, 30, 33, 34). The life circumstances of individuals dictate their choices, their behaviors, and ultimately, their health. For example, certain urban areas in which a large percentage of the residents are Black and poor have fewer grocery stores with healthy, fresh foods and greater exposure to environmental hazards (such as air pollution). These life circumstances, and not individual choices, contribute to diminished health among the residents (12).

Social factors, in this context, can be viewed as forces that negatively impact health (12, 29, 35). Achieving equity in health will require eliminating social stressors (circumstances that cause worry or concern (36–38)), including racial discrimination, poverty, and insecurity surrounding food, economic well-being, employment, neighborhood, and housing (36–38). Such factors contribute to creating inequities in health.

The recognition of the importance of social factors as determinants of health led to an emphasis in Healthy People 2020 (39) and Healthy People 2030 (40) on addressing social determinants of health to improve public, community, and individual health. Social, economic, environmental, political, and other factors have been identified as overall playing a greater role in health than individual risk factors or behaviors (12) or health care.

Several models have been developed to identify Social Determinants of Health (SDOH). The most widely used model of SDOH was developed by the CDC (29).

The CDC defines SDOH as the conditions in which people live, work, learn, and play. These factors in the social, political, and physical environment have significant impacts upon human health. They are often determined by political and economic policies (42).

Overall, the body of research about health inequities is focused upon a constellation of factors in the social and physical environment that exert a negative influence upon health. These factors include:

- Exposure to chronic, ongoing psychosocial stressors including racial discrimination, family relationships, family illness and death, and legal problems within the family;
- Economic instability and poverty;
- Unemployment and work instability;
- Housing instability, crowding, and poor housing conditions;
- Neighborhood conditions such as crime, violence, policing, lack of access to healthy food, lack of green spaces for exercise and relaxation, and environmental toxins;
- Lack of early childhood education programs, poor-quality schools;
- Lack of transportation;
- Lack of access to appropriate, accessible, good-quality health care.

The five major Social Determinants of Health included in the CDC model are:

Social and community context;
Access to education and quality of education;

Economic stability;
Neighborhood and built environment;
Access to and quality of health care.

(29)

These five factors from the CDC model of SDOH are discussed in the following paragraphs.

Social and community context refers to the social aspects of family, neighborhood, and community life. The social and community aspects of life are at the heart of Social Determinants of Health. The characteristics of family and community life, often termed the "social environment," are important determinants of health (43, 44).

Decades of research have shown that overall, as identified by pioneers in Social Epidemiology such as Drs. John Cassell, Leonard Syme, George Caplan, Lisa Berkman, Sherman James, David Williams, Nancy Krieger, Arline Geronimus, Steven Woolf, Sandro Galea, and others, the social environment has a profound impact upon health (42–44). Factors such as racial discrimination, poverty, and instability in employment, family relationships, health, and housing contribute to poor health (34, 36, 37). Such social stressors are chronic, toxic, uncontrollable, and unpredictable, and cause worry and concern (36, 37). Exposure to such stressors in the social environment has a negative influence upon health.

An important aspect of the social context of lives of Black women is exposure to chronic, ongoing, social stressors, such as discrimination based upon race or gender. "Psychosocial stressors," in this context, are problems or circumstances of life that create chronic worry, concern, fear, or anxiety (36, 37). The pandemic of COVID-19 has been described as creating a "pandemic of stress," due to the harmful stressors created by the pandemic, such as deterioration of physical and mental health, job loss and economic decline, and severe illness and deaths in families (45). Widespread racial discrimination faced by Black women enhances the harmful impact of exposure to chronic social stressors.

Racism has been termed a "public health crisis" by the Robert Wood Johnson Foundation (46), due to its significant negative impacts upon health. It is a major source of exposure to stressors in the social environment of young Black women and has been identified as an important underlying cause of racial inequities in health (34, 42).

"Racism" refers to unfair, unjust, or discriminatory treatment of an individual based upon his or her membership in a minority racial/ethnic group (47). Racism can be interpersonal (directed at an individual) or structural. "Structural racism" refers to unfair, unjust, or discriminatory treatment of members of racial/ethnic minority groups that are embedded in laws, policies, or practices (48). "Structural racism" includes policies, laws, and practices that are deeply rooted in society (such as discriminatory lending practices, which deny Blacks the means to buy homes and thereby acquire wealth (48)). Other examples of structural racism include discriminatory arrest and sentencing practices, which are biased against Blacks. Structural racism is embedded in American society. A more recent term, "Cultural racism," refers to negative stereotypes, beliefs, and attitudes that members of one group use to describe or discriminate against members of another group (34, 49). These negative stereotypes and beliefs can be implicit or explicit. They can become cultural "norms" and impact the treatment of Black women. It has been noted that racial discrimination has existed for so long in the United States and is so pervasive that many Americans have become accustomed to inequality (50). Racism is a major form of chronic social stressors faced by Black women and, as noted previously, is a cause of inequities in health between young Black and White women (42, 50).

Decades of research has demonstrated that ongoing, chronic exposure to the deleterious impact of stressors creates wear and tear upon multiple systems of the body. Beginning in the early 1900s, pioneering researcher Walter B. Cannon wrote in *Bodily Changes in Pain, Hunger, Fear and Rage* that a series of physiologic changes accompanies exposure to stressful events or conditions (51). Hans Selye, another pioneer in research about exposure to stressors, described in *The Stress of Life* (52) the cascade of hormonal changes that accompany exposure to stressors. Later, researchers used the expression "flight or fight" response to describe the changes in the body that accompany exposure to stressful life conditions. The body prepares to run (e.g., to avoid being attacked by an animal) or fight (to defend oneself). While these physiologic changes, mediated by the autonomic nervous system and including increased heart rate and blood pressure and the release of glucose, helped early man to survive, they can have a harmful impact upon human health in the modern world. Chronic exposure to stressors in the social environment can be associated with hypertension and other diseases and can also be associated with markers of inflammation (such as cortisol, released by the adrenal gland, also as part of the stress response), which may increase susceptibility to disease. Many of these negative health effects worsen as Black women age, creating a circumstance termed "weathering" (53, 54), which causes the health of Black women to deteriorate as they age. Moreover, the disparities in health between Black and White women increase with age, due to the premature aging caused by years of exposure to stressful life conditions. Weathering has been suggested as an explanation for the worsening of pregnancy outcomes, such as preterm birth, as Black women age prematurely during their twenties and into their thirties (53, 54). Exposure to chronic stressors causes premature aging in Black compared to White women. One author noted, "One cost of health inequality has been the lives of Black women" (19).

Discrimination exerts a double toll upon Black women, who are victims of discrimination based upon both race and gender. Thoits noted that discrimination based upon race and gender creates a large burden upon Black women when added to other chronic stressors in their lives, such as economic worries and concerns (55).

The roots of racial discrimination in the United States can be traced back to the 1600s, when Blacks were forcibly transported from Africa to the United States as slaves, a historical event termed the "African Diaspora." For centuries, Blacks in the United States were considered as property of their owners. Even those Blacks who were not slaves had few legal rights (e.g., to vote) and faced segregation that denied them access to, for example, public rest rooms and water fountains.

Blacks have been subjected to discriminatory policies and behaviors in the United States for centuries. The development of the Civil Rights Movement after 1950 and the emergence of prominent leaders of this Movement such as the Rev. Martin Luther King, Jr., Malcolm X, Rosa Parks, and John Lewis led to the passage of laws such as the Voting Rights Act and the Civil Rights Act in the 1960s. However, racism continues to exist and to be a significant source of stress and to limit opportunities for Black women. The murders of Black men cause mothers to worry when their sons and other male family members leave their homes and neighborhoods because they may be the victims of unjustified violence or fatal attacks.

Research about the large disparities between Black and White women in poor pregnancy outcomes such as preterm birth (birth at less than 37 weeks of completed gestation) and maternal mortality (death of a woman from causes related to pregnancy and childbirth) (to be discussed in detail in Chapter 3) has focused upon the importance of exposure to chronic psychosocial stressors as increasing the risk of pregnant Black women for these harmful outcomes (36–38). Such stressors include loss of employment, family illness, insufficient financial resources, housing instability, and divorce or separation (36, 37). An analysis of data from the Pregnancy Risk Assessment Monitoring System (PRAMS) of the CDC demonstrated that in 2010, in the year prior to giving birth, Black women of childbearing age had greater exposure to stressful life circumstances than their White counterparts (56). These stressors included problems with finances and their relationship with their partners (56).

In summary, the social, family, neighborhood, job, and community context or environment in which Black women live and work can exert profound harmful impacts upon their health. These impacts can be very deleterious to their health, as occurs with exposure to stressors such as racism, separation and divorce, family illness, economic, employment, and housing instability, and disorganization, crime, and instability in the community or neighborhood (36, 37, 57). Exposure to these chronic stressors in the social environment is associated with premature aging, and physical and mental health problems.

Economic Stability

Poverty, or lack of economic stability, has a negative impact upon health (59–63). The poverty rate among Black women in the United States in 2019 was 22.5 percent. Among White women, the poverty rate in 2019 was 9 percent (59, 60). In other words, a Black woman is more than twice as likely as a White woman to be poor. (In 2021, the poverty level for an individual was defined as an annual income of less than $12,880.00, and for a family of four, poverty was an annual income of less than $26,500.00.)

Poverty frequently occurs concentrated in areas and occurs in families and neighborhoods over long periods of time. In poor communities, the residents have less access to resources to achieve health, such as grocery stores with fresh, healthy foods, and safe neighborhoods. In addition, low-income communities often lack sufficient educational and employment opportunities, perpetuating poverty. Children raised in poor neighborhoods often are poor as adults (40).

Black women also have a greater risk than White women of unemployment and have less wealth than their White counterparts. Poverty therefore often passes from one generation to the next among poor, Black families. Wealth provides access to educational attainment, better quality and stable housing, and financial security. However, the net worth of Whites is about 15 times that of Blacks in the United States (61, 62).

In addition to having less wealth than White women, Black women earn less than White women. Even at higher levels of education (master's degree or professional degree), there are differences in mean annual earnings, with Black women earning less than White women with the same level of education (40). Income inequality between Blacks and Whites has grown in recent decades (61, 62).

Poverty affects health status. One of the most robust findings of Social Epidemiology is the association between poverty and health. According to findings from the National Health Interview Survey (of the National Center for Health Statistics), during the period from 2014 to 2016, poor persons had worse self-reported health than the nonpoor (64). Similarly, in the nine-year follow-up of mortality among adults living in Alameda County, California, the poor had an increased risk of multiple causes of death compared to those who were not poor (65, 66). The Whitehall Study of British civil servants demonstrated diminished health among workers in the lower pay grades than among those earning greater incomes (67).

Low-income women who were pregnant or mothers of young children identified worries about having sufficient funds to pay their bills as a significant source of exposure to stressors (36, 37).

Several factors can help to explain the association between poverty and health. The poor often work at riskier jobs, which may lead to injuries or disability. Their jobs may not provide time to receive health care. They may also have diminished access to health care, as clearly demonstrated by the COVID-19 pandemic. In addition, poor health often restricts the ability of individuals to work, so that poor health may contribute to poverty.

The poor may also have employment and housing instability, a source of chronic stressors. They may often suffer from food insecurity. The absence of stable income, housing, employment, and nutritious food have negative impacts upon health. Recent research found that exposure to poverty during the prenatal period and early childhood years may have a negative impact on the development of a child's brain (68).

In summary, Black women are more likely to be poor than White women. Poverty, in turn, has a negative impact on a wide and diverse array of health risks and outcomes.

Education Access and Quality

Hundreds of studies have been published about the associations between education and health (69). Education is a primary pathway in the United States for the achievement of financial security, stable employment, income, wealth, and safe neighborhoods. Education also impacts access to health care and health literacy (69). Yet, Blacks often lack access to equal educational attainment, due to the schools in the neighborhoods in which they live. For example, local property taxes are used to fund public schools. In neighborhoods with lower property values, in which many Black children live, schools have lower levels of funding for books, teachers, computers, materials, etc. Policy decisions about school budgets, construction, and resources, impact health. Policies about zoning, school districting, school budgets, and construction need to be linked to public health, since these educational issues affect the short-term and long-term health of students.

Education promotes the acquisition of many skills and abilities that are associated with health, such as problem-solving, reaction to stressors, and health literacy (69). Education also promotes the development of social networks, which may help individuals to obtain employment, friends, and spouses. Individuals with higher levels of education have access to homes in better neighborhoods, and these neighborhoods often have access to green spaces for exercise and relaxation, and sources of healthy, fresh foods. These neighborhoods also have less crime and violence, less crowded housing, and fewer environmental toxins.

Neighborhoods

Many characteristics of neighborhoods can be harmful to health. These characteristics include high levels of crowding, crime, litter, pollution, divorce, incarceration, and violence (57, 58). Such neighborhood stressors can give residents a sense of chronic instability and anxiety. Residents experience fear of crime and violence.

In addition, many neighborhoods lack adequate access to grocery stores with fresh, healthy foods, to transportation, and to green spaces for shade, relaxation, and recreation. Healthy foods, transportation, and green spaces are all necessary to promote health. Urban planning decisions need to be made with consideration of the health aspects of neighborhoods and communities.

Several prior studies have found associations between living in areas with indicators of high levels of social instability (incarceration, divorce, crime, and violence) with deleterious health outcomes such as stroke or hypertension (57, 58). Blacks are more likely than Whites to live in such neighborhoods, which has a negative impact upon the health of Black women.

Housing segregation continues to exist in the United States, with low-income Blacks more likely than Whites to live in areas of concentrated poverty and lack of certain resources. Historically, many neighborhoods developed high concentrations of Blacks and poverty due to a policy initiated in the 1930s termed "redlining" (70, 71). Redlining was a Federal policy instituted by the Home Owners' Loan Corporation, which denied loans to purchase homes in certain neighborhoods. Home loans were denied in certain neighborhoods due to the high concentration of residents who were Black or poor. These neighborhoods were deemed to be poor risks for credit due to high concentrations of poor persons, Blacks, and foreign-born individuals. Despite being outlawed in the late 1960s, redlining exerted long-lasting impacts on neighborhood social, demographic, economic, and environmental composition. Many neighborhoods were segregated due to the history of "red-lining," and racial and economic segregation still define these neighborhoods. Recent research has demonstrated that residents of neighborhoods with a history of redlining have increased risk of several harmful health outcomes, such as preterm birth (70) or cancer diagnosed at later stages (71).

Moreover, segregated neighborhoods may have overcrowded housing with greater exposure to pollution than neighborhoods in which Whites live. Discriminatory lending and rental practices, part of systemic racism, place unjust limits on where Black families can live. Some neighborhoods still have high levels of lead in the soil and dust. The lead enters the home of residents (as dust) and can harm young children who ingest it. The lead in dust can collect on toys, floors, window sills, and furniture, and can harm the health and development of young children who ingest lead in dust from their toys and hands (72, 73).

Recent research demonstrated that in many large urban areas of the United States, those persons living in the poorest communities and in communities with the largest concentrations of members of minority groups (based on Census information) have the greatest burden of air pollution from nitrogen dioxide (74). Neighborhood poverty was defined as areas (census tracts) in which greater than one-fifth of households had incomes below the poverty level. These areas had greater levels of pollution than wealthier areas. The poorer areas contributed the least to air pollution, because the residents owned fewer cars and did less driving. The poorer areas also had a disproportionate burden of chronic health problems. Improving the health of residents in these communities will necessitate changing policies that impact poverty, housing, and air quality. Changing health-related behaviors of residents will not result in substantial improvements in health in these low-income minority communities. Efforts "upstream" to change policies related to pollution, air quality, and housing quality are required to create reductions in health disparities.

Access to and Quality of Health Care

Many health problems are attributable to the life circumstances of individuals, and not to access or use of health care. Preventing many health problems can best be achieved by improving the life circumstances of individuals, and not by providing health care or medical interventions. Working "upstream" to change policies, laws, and practices that negatively impact the health of young Black women will have the greatest impact upon improving health outcomes. As noted elsewhere in this book, health care is estimated to be associated with only 10–20 percent of health outcomes in the United States (31).

Despite this, health care is necessary to allow persons with illness to become as healthy as possible. However, various factors limit low-income Black women from having adequate access to health care. These factors, discussed in Chapter 10, include lack of time away from work to see a physician, lack of dependable transportation, lack of health insurance, lack of providers of health care in certain areas (e.g., rural areas), and mistrust of the health care system by many young Black women (caused by many factors, including implicit racism by providers of health care (75)).

Several aspects of health care can have important influences upon health, especially among disadvantaged communities. First, individuals need to be able to receive necessary health care, including primary and preventive care. Access to such care can prevent symptoms and signs of illness (e.g., elevated blood pressure) from worsening and leading to significant or serious disorders such as stroke. Some have suggested that all people need a "medical home," where they can receive comprehensive, coordinated, culturally appropriate, and preventive health care (76, 77).

Trust in the health care system, including physicians, nurses, and hospitals, has been eroded among the Black community in many parts of the United States. This has been caused by a variety of historical events (such as the Tuskegee Study), as well as personal experiences and observations of racism within health care settings. For example, until fairly recently, almost all physicians were White and male. Racist attitudes toward Black women among White, male physicians created an atmosphere of mistrust and discomfort that discouraged Black women from seeking needed health care (78–81).

In addition, the complaints of Black women, especially during pregnancy and the postpartum period (see Chapter 3), are often dismissed or ignored by physicians. This can lead to the development of serious consequences, such as stillbirth or maternal death (78, 79). The lack of respect for the reports of symptoms by Black women adds to mistrust of the health care system.

Young Black women are in need of access to prenatal care during pregnancy, to promote a healthy outcome for the baby and mother. Receipt of early and adequate prenatal care can help to prevent harmful outcomes of pregnancy, such as preterm birth (birth at less than 37 completed weeks of gestation) and low birthweight (weight at birth of 2,500 grams or 5.5 pounds or less). In addition, prior to becoming pregnant, women need primary and preventive care. Prior research has demonstrated that women with pre-existing health conditions when they become pregnant have an increased risk of a poor pregnancy outcome (82, 83). In addition, supplementation with folic acid and other vitamins can promote a healthy pregnancy. It is also recommended that pregnant and postpartum women be screened for depression and referred for treatment if necessary (84). Depression can have deleterious effects on the outcome of a woman's pregnancy (85, 86) and on the health of a woman and her children (see Chapter 8).

Further, women need access to contraception to prevent unintended or unwanted pregnancies. Women with unintended or unwanted pregnancies have an increased risk of a poor pregnancy outcome (such as preterm birth) compared to women with wanted pregnancies (87).

As will be discussed in Chapter 3, Black women have a much greater risk than White women of unintended pregnancy, preterm birth, low birthweight, infant mortality, fetal death, maternal mortality, and severe maternal morbidity. The receipt of adequate reproductive health care is necessary to improve poor pregnancy outcomes among Black women.

Summary Comments About Social Determinants of Health

The Social Determinants of Health approach recognizes that the determinants of health for the most part are outside of the health care system and are also not a function of individual behaviors. Rather, social, political, environmental, and economic circumstances create situations that make members of disadvantaged or marginalized groups more vulnerable to health problems.

Taken together, the various aspects of the social environment, described as Social Determinants of Health, such as the social and community context of life, exposure to chronic, stressful life conditions (including racial discrimination), and lack of economic stability, can create feelings of hopelessness and vulnerability, and lack of stability or predictability in life. Overall, the focus of Social Determinants of Health is on the negative impact of aspects of the social environment upon health.

However, as noted by Cassell, Kaplan, and others, the social environment also has positive components (43, 88). These include social support, programs to strengthen women and families, and other health-enhancing resources. These health-enhancing resources can provide young Black women with hope, resilience, and a sense of stability.

Social support can be emotional or instrumental. "Emotional support" is information from family members, friends, neighbors, and co-workers that an individual is loved and valued. "Instrumental support" is tangible aid or help, for example, providing help with transportation or childcare, lending money, or providing assistance with household chores when needed. Both emotional and instrumental supports have positive effects upon health (89).

Thoits and others have reported that social ties and social support can improve physical and mental health (90). Social support can mitigate the impact of exposure to stressors upon health (88–93).

In addition, programs that provide support to young mothers, such as home visitation by nurses or community-based workers, or a primary care "medical home," can be health enhancing. For decades, Olds and others have demonstrated that home visitation or even telephone contact by nurses with new mothers can improve health outcomes for children and mothers (94–97). Other programs have demonstrated that comprehensive, coordinated services for women in one place (e.g., community health centers) can have health-enhancing effects on women. For example, enrollment and attendance at Community Health Centers has been shown to reduce preterm birth outcomes (98).

Part of improving the health of Black women of reproductive age and reducing health inequities includes not only reducing the negative aspects of the social environment (such as exposure to chronic stressors) but also strengthening health-enhancing factors. This includes increased investment in support for programs to benefit women.

Life expectancy at birth decreased around the world as a result of the pandemic of COVID-19. The decrease in life expectancy at birth was worse in the United States than in many other high-income nations. Overall, the United States has worse health than many other high-resource nations. The United States spends more per capita on health care than many other nations but less on social services and social resources. Despite the larger per capita expenditures on health care, citizens of the United States have poorer health and shorter lives than those of other high-resource nations (28). American citizens need to decide if it is acceptable to have poorer health, or if the time has arrived to initiate social, economic, and political policies and programs to become a healthier nation (31). A large part of the needed changes will necessitate addressing health inequities among those populations that bear a disproportionate burden of poor health, such as young Black women.

Focus of This Book

Both the CDC and the Robert Wood Johnson Foundation have noted that in order to fix a problem such as racial disparities in health, it is necessary to **identify and measure** the disparities and to **make injustice visible.** The Robert Wood Johnson Foundation specifically noted, "It is impossible to fix what isn't measured" (99). The approach of Public Health to creating the conditions for people to be healthy involves first defining and measuring health problems (12). Analyses of accurate data need to be available in order to facilitate an improved understanding of health inequities (42). Data have been termed the "building blocks" to enhance understanding of and mitigate health disparities (100).

One of the primary objectives of this book is to show the magnitude, history, and causes of disparities in health between young (reproductive age) Black compared to White women. By making the problems more visible, it will be possible to focus on the injustices and circumstances that create diminished health among Black compared to White women of reproductive age. The focus upon younger women was chosen because in recent years (even prior to the COVID-19 pandemic), the health of Americans during the years before age 50 has been notably deteriorating overall. This is particularly true for Black women. The loss of young Black women is tragic for children, spouses, parents, family members, neighbors, friends, and others. Children, in particular, are negatively impacted by the loss of their mother, who is usually their primary caregiver. The loss of a mother will often create mental health problems for a lifetime for a child (101). Illness and death of parents and grandparents due to COVID-19 may create a generation of children, especially Black children, with long-term harm to mental health.

By identifying, measuring, understanding, and eliminating racial disparities in health between young Black and White women, it will be possible to improve the lives of Black women, children, families, and communities.

Dr. David Satcher, former Surgeon General of the United States, noted, "Reducing and eliminating disparities in health is a matter of life and death. Each year in the United States, thousands of individuals die unnecessarily from easily preventable diseases and conditions" (12). It is crucial for the health of our nation to address inequities in health and disease prevention, and to prioritize the health of vulnerable communities. As Satcher noted, "We all have a role to play."

References

1 Malcolm X, Speech, Los Angeles, California, May 22, 1962.

2 Grooms J, Ortega A, Rubelcaba JA. *The COVID-19 Public Health and Economic Crises Leave Vulnerable Populations Exposed*. Washington, DC: Brookings Institution, August 13, 2020.

3 Kinder M, Ford TN. *Black Essential Workers Lives Matter. They Deserve Real Change, Not Just Lip Service*. Washington, DC: Brookings Institution, June 24, 2020.

4 Kinder M. *Essential But Undervalued: Millions of Health Care Workers Aren't Getting the Pay or Respect They Deserve in the COVID-19 Pandemic*. Washington, DC: Brookings Institution, May 28, 2020.

5 Grace D, Johnson C, Reid T. Racial inequality and COVID-19. *Greenlining*, May 4, 2020.

6 Johnson A, Buford T. Early data shows African Americans have contracted and died of Coronavirus at an alarming rate. *ProPublica*, April 5, 2020.

7 Rushovich T, Boulican M, Chen JT, et al. Sex disparities in COVID-19 mortality vary across U.S. racial groups. *J Gen Internal Med* 2021; 36: 1696–1701.

8 Frye J. *On the Frontlines at Work and at Home: The Disproportionate Effects of the Coronavirus Pandemic on Women of Color*. Washington, DC: Center for American Progress, April 23, 2020.
9 Thebault R, Tran A, Williams DR. The coronavirus is infecting Black Americans at an alarmingly high rate. *Washington Post*, April 17, 2020.
10 Luck AN, Preston SH, Elo IT, Stokes AC. The unequal burden of the COVID-19 pandemic: capturing racial/ethnic disparities in U.S. cause-specific mortality. *SSM Popul Health* 2022; 17: 101012.
11 Galea S, Abdella SM. COVID-19 pandemic, unemployment, and civil unrest underlying deep racial and socioeconomic divides. *JAMA* 2020; 324: 227–228.
12 Satcher D, Higginbotham EJ. The public health approach to eliminating disparities in health. *Am J Public Health* 2008; 98 (Suppl): S8–S11.
13 Williams DR, Costa MV, Odunlami AO, Mohammed SA. Moving upstream: how interventions that address the Social Determinants of Health can improve health and racial disparities. *J Public Health Manag Pract* 2008; 14 (Suppl): S8–S17.
14 Woolf SH, Johnson RE, Fryer GE, et al. The health impact of resolving racial disparities: an analysis of U.S. mortality data. *Am J Public Health* 2004; 94: 2078–2081.
15 Braveman P, Egerter S, Williams DR. The social determinants of health: coming of age. *Ann Rev Public Health* 2011; 32: 381–398.
16 Galea S, Tracy M, Hoggert KJ. Estimated deaths attributable to social factors in the United States. *Am J Public Health* 2011; 101: 1456–1465.
17 Woolf SH. Excess deaths will continue in the United States until the root causes are addressed. *Health Aff* 2022; 41: 1562–1564.
18 Williams DR, Lawrence JA, Davis BA. Racism and health: evidence and needed research. *Ann Rev Public Health* 2019; 40: 105–125.
19 Chinn JJ, Martin IK, Redmond N. Health equity among Black women in the U.S. *J Womens Health* 2021; 30: 212–219.
20 Office of Minority Health. *Data and Profiles: Population Profiles, Black/African American Health*. Washington, DC: United States Department of Health and Human Services, 2023.
21 *Health Disparities and Pregnancy*. Arlington, VA: March of Dimes, June 2021.
22 Healthy people 2010: understanding and improving health, *Final Review*. Hyattsville, MD: Centers for Disease Control and Prevention, National Center for Health Statistics, 2012.
23 Williams DR, Purdue-Vaughns V. Needed interventions to reduce racial/ethnic disparities in health. *J Health Politics, Policy Law* 2016; 41: 627–651.
24 Lavisso-Mourey RJ, Besser RE, Williams DR. Understanding and mitigating health inequities – past, present, and future. *NEJM* 2021; 384: 1681–1684.
25 Braveman P, Gottleib L. The social determinants of health: it's time to consider the causes of the causes. *Public Health Rep*. 2014; 129 (Suppl 2): 19–31.
26 Woolf SH. *Social and Economic Policies Can Help to Reverse Americans' Declining Health*. Washington, DC: Center for American Progress, September, 2021.
27 Yong E. America was in an early death crisis long before COVID. *The Atlantic*, July 23, 2022.
28 Woolf SH, Aron L (eds). National research council, commission on population. In *United States Health in International Perspective: Shorter Lives, Poorer Health*. Washington, DC: National Academies Press, 2013.
29 Hacker K, Auerbach J, Iked R, et al. Social determinants of health: an approach taken at CDC. *J Public Health Manag Pract* 2022; 28: 589–594.

30 Woolf SH. Social and economic policies can help to reverse Americans' declining health. *Am J Prev Med* 2004; 27: 49–56.
31 Weintraub K. Americans' life expectancy continues to fall, erasing health gains of the last quarter century. *USA Today*, December 22, 2022.
32 *Report of the Secretary's Task Force on Black and Minority Health (Heckler Report)*. Washington, DC: United States Department of Health and Human Services, 1985.
33 Miller CA. Societal change and public health: a rediscovery. *Am J Public Health* 1976; 66: 54–60.
34 Williams DR, Lawrence JA, Davis BA, Vu C. Understanding how discrimination can affect health. *Health Serv Res* 2019; 54 (Suppl 2): 1374–1388.
35 American Public Health Association. Structural racism is a public health crisis: impact on the Black community. *APHA Policy Statement Number LB20–04*, October 24, 2020.
36 Orr ST, James SA, Charney E. A social environment inventory for the pediatric office. *J Dev Behav Pediatr* 1989; 10: 287–291.
37 Orr ST, James SA, Casper R. Psychosocial stressors and low birthweight: development of a questionnaire. *J Dev Behav Pediatr* 1992; 13: 343–347.
38 Orr ST, James SA, Miller CA, et al. Psychosocial stressors and low birthweight in an urban population. *Am J Prev Med* 1996; 12: 450–466.
39 *Healthy People 2020*. Hyattsville, MD: Office of Disease Prevention and Health Promotion, United States Department of Health and Human Services, 2021.
40 Healthy People 2030. *Building a Healthy Future for All*. Hyattsville, MD: Office of Disease Prevention and Health Promotion, United States Department of Health and Human Services, 2022.
41 Thornton R, Glover C, Cene C, et al. Evaluating strategies for reducing health disparities by addressing the social determinants of health. *Health Aff* 2016; 35: 1416–1423.
42 James SA. Confronting the moral economy of United States racial/ethnic health disparities. *Am J Public Health* 2002; 93: 189.
43 Cassel J. The contribution of the social environment to host resistance. *Am J Epidemiol* 1976; 104: 107–123.
44 Syme SL. The social environment and health. *Daedalus* 1994; 123: 79–86.
45 Williams DR. Stress was already killing Black Americans- COVID-19 is making it worse. *Washington Post*, May 13, 2020.
46 Williams DR. *Why Discrimination Is a Health Issue*. Princeton, NJ: Robert Wood Johnson Foundation, May 26, 2021.
47 *Cancer Facts and Figures for African American/Black People, 2022–2024*. Atlanta, GA: American Cancer Society, 2022.
48 Braveman P, Arkin E, Proctor D, et al. Systemic and structural racism: definitions, examples, health damages, and approaches to dismantling. *Health Aff* 2022; 41: 171–178.
49 Cogburn C. Culture, race, and health: implications for racial inequities and population health. *Milbank Q* 2019; 97: 736–761.
50 Koh HK. The COVID-19 pandemic shows why we must- and how we can- end racial injustice in health. *Time*, June 18, 2020.
51 Cannon WB. *Bodily Changes in Pain, Hunger, Fear, and Rage*. New York: D. Appleton and Co., 1929.
52 Selye H. *The Stress of Life*. New York: McGraw-Hill, 1956.

53 Geronimus AT, Hicken M, Keene D, Bound J. Weathering and age patterns of allostatic load among blacks and whites in the United States. *Am J Public Health* 2006; 96: 826–833.
54 Geronimus AT. Understanding and eliminating racial inequalities in women's health in the United States: the role of the weathering conceptual framework. *J Am Med Womens Assoc* 2001; 56: 133–136.
55 Thoits P. Gender and race stress and health: major findings and policy implications. *J Health Soc Behav* 2010; 51 (Suppl): S41–S53.
56 Burns ER, Farr SI, Howards PP. Stressful life events experienced by women in the year before their infants' births – United States, 2000–2010. *Morb Mortal Wkly Rep* 2015; 64: 247–251.
57 Harburg E, Erfurt JC, Chapel C, et al. Socioecologic stress areas and black-white blood pressure: Detroit. *J Chronic Dis.* 1973; 26: 595–611.
58 James SA, Kleinbaum DG. Socioecologic stress and hypertension-related mortality rates in North Carolina. *Am J Public Health* 1976; 66: 354–358.
59 Bleiweis R, Boesch D, Gaines AC. *The Basic Facts about Women in Poverty.* Washington, DC: Center for American Progress, August 3, 2020.
60 Ross K, Dora Z. *The Latent Poverty, Income, and Food Insecurity Data Reveal Continuing Racial Disparities.* Washington, DC: Center for American Progress, December 21, 2022.
61 Chetty R, Hendren N, Jones MR, Porter SR. Race and economic opportunity in the United States: an intergenerational perspective. *Q J Econ* 2020; 135: 711–783.
62 Chetty R, Hendren N, Katz LP. The effects of exposure to better neighborhoods on children: new evidence from the moving to opportunity experiment. *Am Econ Rev* 2016; 106: 855–902.
63 Woolf SH, Johnson RE, Geiger HJ. The rising prevalence of severe poverty in America: a growing threat to public health. *Am J Prev Med* 2006; 31: 332–341.
64 Braveman PA, Cubbin C, Egeter S, et al. Socioeconomic disparities in health in the United States: what the patterns tell us. *Am J Public Health* 2010; 100 (Suppl 1): S186–S196.
65 Haan M, Caplan G, Camacho T. Poverty and health: prospective evidence from the Alameda County Study. *Am J Epidemiol* 1987; 125: 989–998.
66 Berkman LF, Breslow L (eds). *Health and Ways of Living.* New York: Oxford University Press, 1983.
67 Marmot M, Smith GD, Stansfield S, et al. Health inequalities among British civil servants: the Whitehall II study. *Lancet* 1991; 337: 1387–1393.
68 Blair C, Raver C. Poverty, stress, and brain development – new directions for prevention and intervention. *Acad Pediatr* 2016; 16 (Suppl 3): S30–S36.
69 Zimmerman E, Woolf SH. Understanding the relationship between education and health. *National Academy of Medicine Discussion Paper*, June 5, 2014.
70 Krieger N, Van Wye G, Huynh M, et al. Structural racism, historical redlining, and risk of preterm birth in New York City, 2013–2017. *Am J Public Health* 2020; 110: 1046–1053.
71 Krieger N, Wright E, Chen JT, et al. Cancer stage at diagnosis, historical redlining, and current neighborhood characteristics: breast, cervical, lung, and colorectal cancers, Massachusetts, 2001–2015. *Am J Epidemiol* 2020; 189: 1065–1075.
72 Charney E, Sayre J, Coulter M. Increased lead absorption in inner city children: where does the lead come from? *Pediatrics* 1980; 65: 226–231.

73 Lanphear BP, Weitzman M, Eberly S. Racial differences in urban children's environmental exposure to lead. *Am J Public Health* 1996; 86: 1460–1463.
74 Fuller G. Poorest areas bear the brunt of air pollution. *The Guardian*, September 9, 2022.
75 Hostetter M, Klein S. *In Focus: Reducing Racial Disparities in Health Care by Confronting Racism*. New York: Commonwealth Fund, September 27, 2018.
76 Starfield B. Access, primary care, and the medical home: rights of passage. *Med Care* 2008; 46: 1015–1016.
77 Starfield B, Shi L. The medical home, access to care, and insurance: a review of the evidence. *Pediatrics* 2004; 113: 1493–1498.
78 Cotton TM. I was pregnant and in crisis and all the doctors saw was an incompetent Black woman. *Time*, January 5, 2019.
79 Eldeib D. She says doctors ignored her concerns about her pregnancy. For many Black women, it's a familiar story. *Pro Publica*, December 27, 2022.
80 Smedley BD, Stith AY, Nelson AR (eds). *Unequal Treatment: Confronting Racial and Ethnic Disparities in Health Care*. Washington, DC: Institute of Medicine, National Academies Press, 2003.
81 Byrd WM, Clayton LA. *Eliminating Racial and Ethnic Disparities in Health Care: Background Paper. Racial and Ethnic Disparities in Health Care – Background and History*. Washington, DC: National Academies Press, 2002.
82 Orr ST, Blackmore-Prince CB, James SA. Race, clinical factors, and pregnancy outcomes in a low-income, urban setting. *Ethn Dis* 2000; 10: 411–417.
83 Goldman D, Smith JP. The increasing value of education to health. *Soc Sci Med* 2011; 72: 1728–1737.
84 Mondez JK, Berkman LF. Trends in the educational gradient of mortality among U.S. adults aged 45–84 years: bringing regional context into the explanation. *Am J Public Health*. 2014; 104: e82–e90.
85 Orr ST, James SA, Prince CB. Maternal prenatal depressive symptoms and spontaneous preterm birth among African American women in Baltimore, Maryland. *Am J Epidemiol* 2002; 156: 797–802.
86 Hoffman S, Hatch MC. Depressive symptomatology during pregnancy: evidence for an association with decreased fetal growth in pregnancies of lower social class women. *Health Psychol* 2000; 19: 535–543.
87 Orr ST, Miller CA, James SA, et al. Unintended pregnancy and preterm birth. *Paediatr Perinat Epidemiol* 2000; 14: 309–313.
88 Kaplan BH, Cassel JC, Gore S. Social support and health. *Med Care* 1977; 15 (Suppl): 147–158.
89 Orr ST. Social support and pregnancy outcome: a review of the literature. *Clin Obstet Gynecol* 2004; 47: 842–855.
90 Thoits PA. Mechanisms linking social ties and support to physical and mental health. *J Health Soc Behav* 2011; 52: 145–161.
91 Broadhead WE, Kaplan BH, James SA, et al. The epidemiologic evidence for a relationship between social support and health. *Am J Epidemiol* 1983; 117: 521–537.
92 Cohen S, Syme SL (eds). *Social Support and Health*. San Francisco: Academic Press, 1985.
93 Nuckolls KB, Kaplan BH, Cassel JC. Psychosocial assets, life crises and the prognosis of pregnancy. *Am J Epidemiol* 1972; 95: 431–441.
94 Olds DL. Prenatal and infancy home visiting by nurses: from randomized trials to community replication. *Prev Sci* 2002; 3: 153–172.

95 Olds DL, Henderson CR, Kitzman H. Prenatal and infancy home visitation by nurses: recent findings. *Future Child.* 1999; 9: 44–65.
96 Olds DL, Donelan-McCall N, O'Brien R, et al. Improving the nurse-family partnership in community practice. *Pediatrics* 2013; 132 (Suppl 2): S110–S117.
97 Olds DL, Kitzman H, Cole RF, et al. Enduring effects of prenatal and infancy home visiting by nurses on maternal life-course and government spending: follow-up of a randomized trial among children at age 12 years. *Arch Pediatr Adolesc Med* 2010; 164: 419–424.
98 Whelan E. *The Importance of Community Health Centers.* Washington, DC: Center for American Progress, August 9, 2010.
99 Hostetetter M, Klein S. *In Focus: Reducing Racial Disparities in Health Care by Confronting Racism.* Washington, DC: Commonwealth Fund, September 27, 2018.

2 Indicators of Mortality

Indicators of Mortality

When considering the health of different groups, it is useful to begin by comparing indicators of mortality between the groups of interest. There are several important measures of mortality that are frequently used to provide an indication of the health of a group (by race, gender, country, etc.) and to compare the health of groups. In this chapter, measures of mortality for young Black women in the United States will be compared to those of young White women.

Life Expectancy at Birth

One of the most widely utilized measures of mortality used to compare the health of groups is life expectancy at birth. Life expectancy is a mathematical average that takes into account the mortality experience of a group over a lifetime. Consequently, infant mortality, childhood mortality, deaths of young adults, etc., are taken into account in calculating life expectancy at birth. Life expectancy at birth provides an indicator of the average number of years a member of a group might be expected to live.

As shown in Table 2.1, in 1900, the life expectancy at birth of White females was 48.7 years, while for Black females, it was 15 years less (33.5 years). By 1950, the gap in life expectancy at birth between Black and White females had decreased to 9.3 years, with White females expected to live on average 72.2 years and Black females, 62.0 years. Life expectancy at birth continued to increase for both Black and White females through 2010, and the disparity between the two groups continued to diminish, as shown in Table 2.1.

Some describe life expectancy as being determined by a combination of policies, social factors, and scientific advances (1–19). This description is based on a recognition that health is largely determined by social and political factors, and not by the behaviors of individuals or factors within the health care system.

DOI:10.4324/9781032663807-2

Table 2.2 shows life expectancy at birth in recent years (2010–2020) for Black and White females. It can be seen in this table that for the years 2014–2016, life expectancy at birth decreased for both White females and Black females. In addition, life expectancy substantially decreased for both groups

Table 2.1 Life Expectancy at Birth for Black and White Females, 1900–2010 (Life Expectancy at Birth in Years)

Year	*White Females*	*Black Females*	*Differences*
1900	48.7	33.5	15.2
1950	72.2	62.9	9.3
1960	74.1	66.3	7.8
1970	75.6	68.3	7.3
1980	78.1	72.5	5.6
1990	79.4	73.6	5.8
1995	79.6	73.9	5.7
2000	79.9	75.1	4.8
2001	80.0	75.3	4.7
2002	80.1	75.4	4.7
2003	80.2	75.7	4.5
2004	80.5	76.1	4.4
2005	80.5	76.2	4.3
2006	80.7	76.7	4.0
2007	80.9	77.0	3.9
2008	80.9	77.3	3.6
2009	81.2	77.7	3.5
2010	81.3	78.0	3.3

Source: (References: 19, 20)

Table 2.2 Life Expectancy at Birth for Black and White Females, 2010–2021 (Life Expectancy in Years)

Year	*White Females*	*Black Females*	*Difference*
2010	81.3	78.0	3.3
2011	81.1	77.8	3.3
2012	81.2	78.1	3.1
2013	81.2	78.1	3.1
2014	81.2	78.2	3
2015	81	78.1	2.9
2016	81	78	3
2017	81	78.1	2.9
2018	81.1	78.1	3
2019	81.3	78.2	3.1
2020	80.2	75.7	4.5
2021	79.2	74.8	4.4

Source: (References: 20–22)

from 2019 to 2020, due largely to the pandemic of COVID-19. The decrease in life expectancy at birth from 2019 to 2020 was -2.4 percent for Black females and -1.1 percent for White females. The difference in life expectancy at birth between Black and White females increased from 3.1 years in 2019 to 4.5 years in 2020. These data suggest that the pandemic had a larger impact on life expectancy at birth for Black than White females but that life expectancy at birth was affected by COVID-19 for both Black and White females. Life expectancy at birth continued to decrease from 2020 to 2021 for Black and White women, as shown in Table 2.2.

Age-Adjusted All-Cause Mortality

Another important indicator of population or group health is age-adjusted all-cause mortality. Age adjustment is necessary because one group may contain proportionately more older persons than another and would be expected to have higher rates of mortality. Age adjustment removes the impact on mortality of having proportionately more older persons in a group.

Table 2.3 shows the age-adjusted all-cause mortality per 100,000 population for Black females and White females for the period 1900 to 2010. For most of this time period, the ratio comparing mortality of Black to White females was approximately 1.3. The age-adjusted all-cause mortality per 100,000 population for both Black females and White females declined substantially from 1900 to 2010, but the ratio of age-adjusted all-cause mortality

Table 2.3 Age-Adjusted All-Cause Mortality per 100,000 Population, Females, by Race, 1900–2010

Year	*Race*		*Ratio BF: WF*
	Black Females	*White Females*	
1900	3,308	2,394	1.38
1910	2,875.3	2,154	1.33
1920	2,756.2	2,025.9	1.36
1930	2,530.1	1,726.6	1.47
1940	2,057.5	1,550.4	1.33
1950	1,574.1	1,198	1.31
1960	1,340.5	1,074.4	1.25
1970	1,228.7	944	1.3
1980	1,033.3	796.1	1.3
1990	975.1	728.8	1.34
2000	927.6	715.3	1.3
2010	898.2	741.8	1.21

Source: (References: 19, 20, 23–25)

Table 2.4 Age-Adjusted All-Cause Mortality, Females, by Race, the United States, 2016–2020

Year	*Race*		*Ratio BF: WF*
	Black Females	*White Females*	
2016	734.1	637.2	1.15
2017	854.1	734.5	1.16
2018	852.9	725.4	1.18
2019	724.9	627.4	1.16
2020	1119	834.7	1.34

Source: (References: 26–28)

for Black females compared to age-adjusted all-cause mortality for White females remained relatively unchanged, at approximately 1.3.

The age-adjusted all-cause mortality for Black females and White females from 2016 to 2020 is shown in Table 2.4. The overall declines in age-adjusted mortality from all causes continued for both White and Black females over this time period, except for increases from 2016 to 2017, and most notably from 2019 to 2020. The increase in age-adjusted mortality from all causes from 2019 to 2020 was +24.9 percent for Black females and +12.1 percent for White females. The large increases for the period 2019 to 2020 are likely attributable to deaths from COVID-19, as well as causes exacerbated by infection with COVID-19, such as heart disease. The ratio comparing age-adjusted mortality rates per 100,000 population for Black: White women also increased from 2019 to 2020, to a level higher than any year since 1930 (26–28).

Table 2.5 shows the age-adjusted mortality for all causes for Black and White females by age group from 1950 to 2019. The women included in this table are all of reproductive age (15 to 44 years). For each time period included, age-adjusted mortality from all causes increased with age for both Black and White females. The ratio of mortality rates comparing Black to White women overall increased with age as well. In other words, the health of Black women, even at relatively young ages, declines with age. This demonstrates support for the "weathering hypothesis" of Geronimus (29). The "weathering hypothesis" suggests that continued exposure to chronic stressful life conditions by Black women during their reproductive years results in diminished health and premature aging over time. In addition, exposure to racism and other social stressors over the life course has a detrimental impact upon health (30–41). Weathering is also associated with increases in health disparities between Black and White women over time.

A recent paper discussed "Missing Americans" (42). This research concluded that approximately one-half of all deaths in 2021 among Americans under age 65 were preventable. The mortality among Americans under age 65 years in 2021 was much greater than the mortality among residents under age 65 of other high-resource (high-income) nations in 2021. The Americans

Table 2.5 Age-Adjusted All-Cause Death Rates per 100,000 Population by Race and Age Among Females, 1950–2019

Year	*Race*	*Age Group*		
		15–24	*25–34*	*35–44*
1950	White Females	71.5	112.8	235.8
	Black Females	213.1	393.3	758.1
	Ratio WF: BF	3	3.49	3.2
1960	White Females	54.9	85	191.1
	Black Females	107.5	273.2	568.5
	Ratio BF: WF	2	3.2	3
1970	White Females	61.6	84.1	193.3
	Black Females	111.9	231	533
	Ratio BF: WF	1.8	2.75	2.8
1980	White Females	55.5	65.4	138.2
	Black Females	70.5	150	323.9
	Ratio BF: WF	1.3	2.3	2.3
1990	White Females	45.9	61.5	117.4
	Black Females	68.7	159.5	298.6
	Ratio BF: WF	1.5	2.6	2.5
2000	White Females	41.1	55.1	125.7
	Black Females	58.3	121.8	271.9
	Ratio BF: WF	1.4	2.2	2.2
2013	White Females	35.5	64.6	126.8
	Black Females	41.2	91	187.9
	Ratio BF: WF	1.2	1.4	1.5
2014	White Females	35.5	66.9	130.7
	Black Females	42.5	88.6	193.9
	Ratio BF: WF	1.2	1.3	1.5
2019	White Females	38.9	86.5	151.6
	Black Females	56.4	111.4	224.3
	Ratio BF: WF	1.45	1.29	1.48

Source: (References: 21, 23–29)

who died prematurely from preventable causes were termed "Missing Americans." These individuals would not have died prematurely if the mortality of Americans less than age 65 were the same as the mortality in other high-resource nations. Blacks are disproportionately represented among "Missing Americans."

Leading Causes of Death

Another way to assess differences in health using data on mortality is to compare age-adjusted deaths overall for the leading causes of death, and separately for each leading cause of death in various age groups by race. Table 2.6 shows the ten leading causes of death for Black and White females aged 20–24 years with the age-adjusted mortality rates for each leading cause and overall (all causes) for 2019 (43). In addition, the ratios of mortality rates comparing Black: White

Table 2.6 Age-Adjusted Mortality Rates for Leading Causes of Death per 100,000 Population, Black and White Females, Ages 20–24 Years, 2019

Black Females, Ages 20–24 Years, Leading Causes of Death and Age-Adjusted Mortality Per 100,000 Population, 2019

Cause of Death	*Mortality Per 100,000 Population*
1. Unintentional Injuries	22.4
2. Homicide	14.2
3. Suicide	5.2
4. Cardiovascular Disease	5.1
5. Cancer	4.2
6. Disorders Related to Pregnancy and Childbirth	2.6
7. Diabetes	1.5
All Causes	73.7

White Females, Ages 20–24 Years, Leading Causes of Death and Age-Adjusted Mortality Per 100,000 Population, 2019

Cause of Death	*Mortality Per 100,000 Population*
1. Unintentional Injuries	23.5
2. Suicide	6.5
3. Cancer	2.8
4. Homicide	2.1
5. Cardiovascular Disease	1.9
6. Congenital Malformations	0.9
7. Disorders Related to Pregnancy and Childbirth	0.9
8. Diabetes	0.6
All Causes	48.7

Selected Ratios BF: WF, Leading Causes of Death, Women Aged 20–24, 2019

All Causes	1.51
Homicide	6.76
Cardiovascular Disease	2.68
Cancer	1.5
Disorders Related to Pregnancy and Childbirth	2.89
Diabetes	2.5

Source: (Reference: 43)

women aged 20–24 years for each leading cause and all causes are shown. Table 2.6 shows that in 2019, the age-adjusted mortality for women aged 20–24 years for all causes was 73.7 per 100,000 for Black females and 48.7 per 100,000 for White females. The ratio comparing age-adjusted mortality from all causes (2019) for Black: White females aged 20–24 years was 1.51.

The second-leading cause of death for Black females aged 20–24 years in 2019 was homicide. As shown in Table 2.6, the age-adjusted mortality from homicide for women aged 20–24 years was 14.2 per 100,000 population for Black females, compared to 2.1 per 100,000 population for White females. The ratio comparing mortality from homicide in 2019 for Black: White women aged 20–24 years was 6.76.

As shown in Table 2.6, other leading causes of mortality in 2019 for which Black females aged 20–24 years had greater age-adjusted mortality included diseases of the heart, malignant neoplasms, disorders related to pregnancy and childbirth, and diabetes mellitus.

The significantly elevated age-adjusted mortality for Black women aged 20–24 years in 2019 from these chronic health conditions places them at increased risk, among other health problems, of poor pregnancy outcomes (44). Prior research has demonstrated that women with chronic health conditions prior to and during pregnancy have increased risk of poor pregnancy outcomes such as preterm birth (see Chapter 3) (44).

Table 2.7 shows the age-adjusted mortality for the ten leading causes of death overall, and separately for each leading cause of death for Black and White females aged 25–34 years for 2019. As shown in Table 2.7, for the ten leading causes of death combined, the age-adjusted mortality per 100,000 population aged 25–34 years was 111.4 for Black females and 86.5 for White females. The ratio comparing Black: White females is 1.29. For both Black and White females aged 25–34 years, the leading cause of death was unintentional injuries, as shown in Table 2.7. For Black females aged 25–34 years, the second-leading cause of death in 2019 was diseases of the heart. Diseases of the heart was the fourth-leading cause of death among White females aged 25–34 years in 2019. The ratio comparing mortality from diseases of the heart for Black: White females aged 25–34 years in 2019 was 2.41. Other leading causes of death for which Black females had significantly elevated age-adjusted mortality rates compared to White females included homicide, disorders related to pregnancy and childbirth, diabetes mellitus, cerebrovascular disease (stroke), and malignant neoplasms (cancer). Black females aged 25–34 years had over four times the age-adjusted mortality rate per 100,000 population for homicide compared to White females in 2019. For other leading causes of death, Black females aged 25–34 years had three times the age-adjusted mortality (disorders related to pregnancy and childbirth, diabetes mellitus) of their White counterparts.

Table 2.8 shows the age-adjusted mortality rates per 100,000 population for the ten leading causes of death overall and for each cause, for Black and White females, aged 35–44 years, 2019. For the ten leading causes of death combined, the age-adjusted mortality per 100,000 population for Black females aged 35–44 years was 224.3, while for White females, it was 151.6. The ratio comparing age-adjusted mortality per 100,000 population for all causes for Black: White females aged 35–44 years was 1.48.

Many of the leading causes of mortality in 2019 are different for Black compared to White females aged 35–44 years. For example, homicide is the

Table 2.7 Age-Adjusted Mortality Rates for Leading Causes of Death per 100,000 Population, Black and White Females, Ages 25–34 Years, 2019

White Females, Ages 25–34 Years, Leading Causes of Death and Death Rates per 100,000 Population	
Cause of Death	*Mortality Per 100,000 Population*
1. Unintentional Injuries	37.2
2. Suicide	8.3
3. Cancer	7.9
4. Cardiovascular Disease	4.9
5. Homicide	2.3
6. Chronic Liver Disease and Cirrhosis	2.1
7. Disorders Related to Pregnancy and Childbirth	1.9
8. Diabetes	1.2
9. Stroke	1.1
10. Influenza and Pneumonia	1
All Causes	86.5
Black Females, Ages 25–34 Years, Leading Causes of Death and Age-Adjusted Mortality Per 100,000 Population, 2019	
Cause of Death	*Mortality Per 100,000 Population*
1. Unintentional Injuries	27.2
2. Cardiovascular Disease	11.8
3. Cancer	10.4
4. Homicide	10
5. Disorders Related to Pregnancy and Childbirth	5.6
6. Suicide	4.6
7. Diabetes	3.5
8. Stroke	2.4
All Causes	111.4
Selected Ratios, BF: WF, Women Aged 25–34, 2019	
All Causes	1.29
Cardiovascular Disease	2.41
Cancer	1.32
Homicide	4.35
Pregnancy and Childbirth	2.95
Diabetes	2.92
Stroke	2.2

Source: (Reference: 43)

fifth-leading cause of death for Black females and the eighth among White females. The ratio comparing age-adjusted mortality per 100,000 women for Black compared to White females for homicide is 3.36. Black females also had considerably greater age-adjusted mortality from diseases of the heart

Table 2.8 Age-Adjusted Mortality Rates for Leading Causes of Death per 100,000 Population, Black and White Females, Ages 35–44 Years, 2019

White Females, Ages 35–44 Years, Leading Causes of Death and Death Rate per 100,000 Population, 2019

Cause of Death	*Mortality per 100,000 Population*
1. Unintentional Injuries	40.3
2. Cancer	29.6
3. Cardiovascular Disease	14.9
4. Suicide	11.4
5. Chronic Liver Disease, Cirrhosis	6.9
6. Diabetes	3.5
7. Stroke	3.2
8. Homicide	2.5
All Causes	151.6

Black Females, Ages 35–44 Years, Leading Causes of Death and Age-Adjusted Mortality Per 100,000 Population, 2019

Cause of Death	*Deaths per 100,000 Population*
1. Cancer	42.2
2. Cardiovascular Disease	38.5
3. Unintentional Injuries	32.5
4. Diabetes	8.7
5. Homicide	8.4
6. Stroke	7.8
7. HIV	5.4
8. Nephritis	5.2
9. Disorders Related to Pregnancy and Childbirth	4.7
10. Suicide	4.3
All Causes	224.3

Selected Ratios BF: WF, Women Aged 35–44, 2019

All Causes	1.48
Cancer	1.43
Cardiovascular Disease	2.58
Diabetes	2.49
Homicide	3.36
Stroke	2.44

Source: (Reference: 43)

(ratio Black: White females = 2.58), cerebrovascular disease (ratio Black: White females = 2.44), diabetes mellitus (ratio Black: White females = 2.49), and malignant neoplasms (ratio Black: White females = 1.43). Mortality from HIV (human immunodeficiency virus) was the seventh-leading cause of death for Black females aged 35–44 years in 2019 but does not appear in the top ten leading causes of death for White females aged 35–44 years.

Social Determinants of Health and Mortality

Based upon data about mortality, even among younger women, Black females have much poorer health than their White counterparts. Many of the deaths are both premature and preventable. Research about the associations between exposure of women to chronic, ongoing social stressors (e.g., racism, poverty) demonstrates that women with higher levels of exposure to chronic stressors have increased risk of poor health and pregnancy outcomes compared to women with lower levels of exposure to chronic stressors (34, 35, 39). Black women are exposed to life stressors by virtue of social, economic, environmental, and political factors that impact their lives and determine many of the circumstances of their lives (45, 46).

The United States has been termed a "Rich Death Trap," due to the harmful combination of exposure to guns, violence, cars, and disease (47). There is a need for the political will to create major changes in the following:

Availability, safety, and storage of guns;
Acceptance of violent behavior, including by police, and often directed at Black men and Black women;
Safety of persons in cars;
Public health infrastructure to protect Americans from diseases.

It is time to demand that both physical security and health security in the United States are addressed and improved (48). This will require investment in public health infrastructure to allow all Americans to achieve the best health possible.

The data presented are for women of reproductive age. The death of these young women, many of whom are mothers, has a devastating impact upon the family. The loss of a mother can affect the mental health of a child for a lifetime (49).

In addition, many women in this age group (ages 20–44 years) are wives, daughters, sisters, friends, and neighbors who fulfill important roles in their families, communities, churches, and places of employment.

Summary

For every indicator of mortality, including life expectancy at birth, age-adjusted all-cause mortality, and leading causes of death, Black women have excess mortality compared to White women. This provides a picture of a population group clearly in poorer health than others. These data support the expression, "Shorter Lives, Poorer Health" (11).

A number of factors in the social environment contribute to these disparities, including exposure to chronic stressful life conditions, racial discrimination, poverty, neighborhood problems (crowding, absence of adequate food stores), and lack of access to health care.

In order to eliminate racial inequities in health, as demonstrated by excess mortality, it will be necessary to measure and understand the social environment in which Black women of reproductive age live. In addition, programs will need to be designed, implemented, and evaluated to improve the social environment of young Black women. This includes both reducing exposure to stressors in the social and physical environment and developing and implementing health-enhancing resources.

As noted by James (51), Woolf et al. (50), Miller (52), and others, there is not a lack of solutions to improve the health of Americans by addressing the Social Determinants of Health. However, the political will to confront racism, poverty, lack of educational and employment opportunities, lack of access to needed health care, and dangerous neighborhood and environmental conditions is missing. As Carratala and Maxwell commented, health inequities do not result from individual behaviors but are the result of "decades of systematic inequality in economic, housing, and health care systems" (18). Carratala and Maxwell also wrote, "Alleviating health disparities will require a deliberate and sustained effort to address social determinants of health, such as segregation, environmental degradation, and racial discrimination" (18).

References

1 Crimmins EM. Lifespan and health-span: past, present, and future. *Gerontologist* 2015; 55: 901–911.
2 Chambie J. One thing Americans can't deny: the nation's low life expectancy. *The Hill*, December 1, 2021.
3 Gutin I, Hummer RA. Social inequality and the future of U.S. life expectancy. *Ann Rev Sociol* 2021; 47: 501–520.
4 Rabin RC. United States life expectancy falls again in "historic" setback. *New York Times*, August 31, 2022.
5 Weintraub K. Americans' life expectancy continues to fall, erasing health gains of the last quarter century. *USA Today*, December 22, 2022.
6 Chetty R, Stepner M, Abraham S, et al. The association between income and life expectancy in the United States, 2001–2014. *JAMA* 2016; 315: 1750–1766.
7 Olshansky SJ, Antonucci T, Berkman LF, et al. Differences in life expectancy due to race and educational differences are widening and many may not catch up. *Health Aff* 2012; 31: 1803–1813.
8 Avendano M, Kawachi I. Why do Americans have shorter life expectancy and worse health than other high-income countries? *Ann Rev Public Health* 2014; 35: 307–325.
9 Rakshit S, McGoug LM, Amin K, Cox C. How does United States life expectancy compare to other countries? *Kaiser Family Foundation: Health System Tracker*, December 6, 2022.

10 Woolf SH, Masters RK, Aron LY. Changes in life expectancy between 2019 and 2020 in the United States and 21 peer countries. *JAMA Netw Open* 2022; 5: e227067.
11 Woolf SH, Aron L (eds). *US Health in International Perspective: Shorter Lives, Poorer Health*. Washington, DC: National Academies Press, 2013.
12 Koh HK, Parekh AK, Park JJ. Confronting the rise and fall of US life expectancy. *JAMA* 2019; 322: 1963–1965.
13 Kuehn BM. US life expectancy lowest since 1996. *JAMA* 2023; 329: 280.
14 Woolf SH, Schoomaker H. Life expectancy and mortality rates in the United States, 1959–2017. *JAMA* 2019; 322: 1996–2016.
15 Chetty R, Stepner M, Abraham S, et al. The association between income and life expectancy in the United States, 2001–2014. *JAMA* 2016; 315: 1750–1766.
16 Brangham W, Coles D. US life expectancy sees "massive decline," especially in black and brown communities. *PBS Newshour*, June 24, 2021.
17 Lavisso-Mourey R, Besser R, Williams DR. Understanding and mitigating health inequities- past, current, and future directions. *NEJM* 2021; 384: 1681–1684.
18 Health United States, 2015. *With Special Feature on Racial and Ethnic Disparities*. Hyattsville, MD: National Center for Health Statistics, 2016.
19 *Health, United States, 2017, with Special Feature on Mortality*. Hyattsville, MD: National Center for Health Statistics, 2018.
20 Arias E, Minino A, Curtin S, Tejada-Vera B. United States decennial life tables, 2009–2011. *National Vital Statistics Reports 69 (8)*. Hyattsville, MD: National Center for Health Statistics, August 7, 2020.
21 *Health United States, 2019*. Hyattsville, MD: National Center for Health Statistics, 2020.
22 Arias E, Tejada-Vera B, Ahmad F, Kochanek KD. Provisional life expectancy estimates for 2020. *Vital Statistics Rapid Release No. 015*. Hyattsville, MD: National Center for Health Statistics, July 2021.
23 Arias E, Tejada-Vera B, Kochanek KD, Ahmad FB. Provisional life expectancy estimates for 2021. *Vital Statistics Rapid Release No. 23*. Hyattsville, MD: National Center for Health Statistics, August 2022.
24 Kochanek KD, Xu J, Arias E. Mortality in the United States, 2019. *Data Brief No. 395*. Hyattsville, MD: National Center for Health Statistics, December 2021.
25 Kochanek KD, Murphy SL, Xu J, Arias E. Mortality in the United States, 2016. *Data Brief No. 293*. Hyattsville, MD: National Center for Health Statistics, December 2017.
26 Xu J, Murphy SL, Kochanek KD, Arias E. Mortality in the United States, 2021. *Data Brief Number 456*. Hyattsville, MD: National Center for Health Statistics, December 2022.
27 Xu J, Arias E. Deaths: final data for 2019. *Vital Statistics Rapid Release, Number 23*. Hyattsville, MD: National Center for Health Statistics, August 2022.
28 Murphy SL, Kochanek KD, Xu J, Arias E. Mortality in the United States, 2020. *Data Brief 427*. Hyattsville, MD: National Center for Health Statistics, December 2021.
29 Geronimus AT. Weathering and age patterns of allostatic load scores among blacks and whites in the United States. *Am J Public Health* 2006; 96: 826–833.
30 Thoits PA. Stress and health: major findings and policy implications. *J Health Soc Behav* 2010; 51 (Suppl): S41–S53.
31 Bailey ZD, Krieger N, Agenor M, et al. Structural racism and health inequities in the USA: evidence and interventions. *Lancet* 2017; 389: 1453–1463.

32 Williams DR, Lawrence JA, Davis BP. Racism and health: evidence and needed research. *Ann Rev Public Health* 2019; 40: 105–125.
33 Orr ST, James SA, Miller CA, et al. Psychosocial stressors and low birthweight in an urban population. *Am J Prev Med* 1996; 12: 459–466.
34 Dole N, Savitz DA, Hertz-Picciotto I, et al. Maternal stress and preterm birth. *Am J Epidemiol* 2003; 157: 14–24.
35 Kasl SV. Stress and health. *Ann Rev Public Health* 1984; 5: 319–341.
36 Cassel J. The contribution of the social environment to host resistance. *Am J Epidemiol* 1976; 104: 107–123.
37 American Public Health Association. Structural racism is a public health crisis: impact on the Black community. *APHA Policy Statement Number LB 20–04*, October 24, 2020.
38 Thoits P. Race and gender stress and health: major findings and policy implications. *J Health Soc Behav* 2010; 51 (Suppl): S41–S53.
39 James SA. Confronting the moral economy of US racial/ethnic health disparities. *Am J Public Health* 2002; 93: 189.
40 Williams DR, Lawrence JA, Davis BA, Vu C. Understanding how discrimination can affect health. *Health Serv Res* 2019; 54 (Suppl 2): 1374–1388.
41 Yong E. America was in an early death crisis long before COVID. *Atlantic*, July 21, 2022.
42 Heron M. Deaths: leading causes for 2019. *National Vital Statistics Reports; 70 (9)*. Hyattsville, MD: National Center for Health Statistics, 2021.
43 Orr ST, Reiter JP, James SA, Orr CA. Maternal health prior to pregnancy and preterm birth among urban, low-income black women in Baltimore: the Baltimore Preterm Birth Study. *Ethn Dis* 2011; 22: 85–89.
44 Orr ST, James SA, Casper R. Psychosocial stressors and low birthweight: development of a questionnaire. *J Dev Behav Pediatr* 1992; 13: 343–347.
45 Orr ST, James SA, Charney E. A social environment inventory for the pediatric office. *J Dev Behav Pediatr* 1989; 10: 287–291.
46 Thompson D. America is a rich death trap. *Atlantic*, September 7, 2022.
47 Nyce CM. The very real lessons America learned from COVID. *Atlantic*, October 17, 2022.
48 Hillis SD, Blenkinsop A, Villaves H, et al. COVID-19 associated orphanhood and caregiver death in the United States. *Pediatrics* 2021; 148: e2021053760.
49 Woolf SH, Johnson RE, Fryer GE, et al. The health impact of resolving racial disparities: an analysis of US mortality data. *Am J Public Health* 2004; 94: 2078–2081.
50 Miller CA. Societal change and public health: a rediscovery. *Am J Public Health* 1976; 66: 54–60.
51 Carratala S, Maxwell C. *Health Disparities by Race and Ethnicity*. Washington, DC: Center for American Progress, May 7, 2020.

3 Pregnancy Outcomes, Infant Mortality, and Maternal Health

Introduction

In the United States, there are large disparities and inequities between Black and White women in poor outcomes related to pregnancy and childbirth, including infant mortality, birth outcomes, and maternal (pregnancy-related) mortality and morbidity. These poor outcomes are of great public health importance. Moreover, these indicators of maternal and child health are worse for the United States than for other high-income countries.

Infant Mortality

One of the most widely used and significant indicators of the health of a population group is infant mortality, which is the number of deaths within the first year of life per 1,000 live births. The United States has one of the highest levels in the world of infant mortality among high-resource nations. Moreover, Blacks have over two times the rate of infant mortality compared to Whites in the United States.

Table 3.1 shows infant mortality for Blacks and Whites in the United States from 1950 to 2021. It can be seen from this table that Black infants have over twice the risk of death in the first year of life compared to White infants. Moreover, the racial disparities between Black and White infant deaths are long-standing and show no signs of improving (1–6).

The ratio comparing infant mortality of Blacks: Whites in 2020 was the largest it has been (2.5) in any prior year since 1950.

The leading causes of infant mortality in the United States are birth defects (congenital anomalies), preterm birth and low birthweight, sudden infant death syndrome (SIDS), unintentional injuries (e.g., suffocation), and maternal pregnancy complications (3–6).

At all ages, Black women have a greater risk of infant mortality compared to White women, as shown in Table 3.2.

Socioeconomic and social factors contribute to the underlying health conditions, which increase risk of infant mortality. A recent study in North Carolina demonstrated that the counties with the greatest levels of food insecurity also had the highest rates of infant mortality (7).

DOI:10.4324/9781032663807-3

Table 3.1 Infant Mortality by Race, United States, 1950–2021

Year	*Infant Deaths per 1,000 Live Births*		
	Whites	*Blacks*	*Ratio Black: White Infants*
1950	26.8	43.9	1.6
1960	22.9	44.3	1.9
1970	17.8	32.6	1.8
1980	11	21.4	1.9
1990	7.6	18	2.4
1999	5.76	14.14	2.45
2000	5.7	13.59	2.38
2005	5.76	13.63	2.37
2010	5.18	11.46	2.21
2015	4.9	11.25	2.3
2018	4.68	10.62	2.27
2019	4.49	10.62	2.37
2020	4	10	2.5
2021	4.7	10.9	2.3

Source: (References: 1–6)

Table 3.2 Infant Mortality by Race and Age of Mother, United States, 2019

Age of Mother	*Race*		
	Black	*White*	*B: W Ratio*
<20 years	12.03	8.3	1.45
20–24 years	10.92	5.94	1.84
25–29 years	10.28	4.49	2.29
30–34 years	10.34	3.56	2.9
35–39 years	10.06	4.02	2.5
40–54 years	12.71	5.03	2.53

Source: (Reference: 3)

Preterm Birth

As noted previously, a leading cause of infant mortality is preterm birth. Preterm birth (birth at less than 37 completed weeks of gestation) is considered a major public health problem in the United States (8). Blacks have a significantly greater risk of preterm birth compared to Whites, as shown in Table 3.3. Moreover, preterm birth increased in the United States from 2016 to 2021 (except for a small decrease from 2019 to 2020), especially among Blacks. The rate of preterm birth in 2021 was higher than that for any year since 2007 (9).

Preventing preterm births is a major public health challenge, especially among Blacks (8). Factors that increase risk of preterm birth include maternal exposure to chronic stressful life conditions, maternal prenatal depression, maternal pregnancy-related anxiety, unintended pregnancy, maternal poor health prior to pregnancy, and chronic health conditions, such as hypertension (10–15). Many of the factors that increase risk of preterm birth occur with greater frequency among Black than White women (16).

Prior research has identified many factors that increase risk of preterm birth, yet prevention of preterm outcomes remains elusive (8). This is due, in part, because many of the factors that are associated with increased risk of preterm birth are "not modifiable at an individual level and are at play long before pregnancy" (17). Pregnancy outcome and infant health are reflections of maternal, family, and community health.

Maternal health is greatly influenced by social, environmental, and economic factors, which are shaped by policies and political decisions. It was noted in one review that exposure to racism and other stressors during a woman's life course impact the outcome of the pregnancy. "Many pregnant bodies simply cannot keep the weight of society at bay for the full 37 to 40 weeks needed to gestate to term" (17). Pregnancy and the health of a pregnant woman are often viewed as a moment in her life, but pregnancy reflects the elements of her entire lifetime that negatively impact her health, such as poverty, racism, and exposure to environmental toxins. Pregnant Black women are disproportionately burdened by many health problems compared to their White counterparts, including preterm birth.

In addition, the reproductive and prenatal care needed for a healthy pregnancy is frequently not available to pregnant Black women. They are

Table 3.3 Preterm Birth by Race, 1981–2021, United States

Percent of Births Preterm (<37 weeks' gestation)			
Year	*Race*		
	White	*Black*	*Ratio Black: White*
1981	7.9	17.3	2.19
1985	8.2	17.8	2.17
1990	8.9	18.8	2.11
1995	9.7	17.7	1.82
2000	10.4	17.4	1.67
2010	10.77	17.12	1.59
2015	9	13.2	1.47
2016	9.04	13.77	1.5
2017	9.06	13.93	1.5
2018	9.09	14.13	1.6
2019	9.26	14.39	1.6
2020	9.1	14.36	1.6
2021	9.49	14.74	1.6

Source: (Reference: 9)

Table 3.4 Weeks of Completed Gestation for Preterm Infants, by Race, 2018

Weeks of Completed Gestation	*Race of Mother*		*B: W Ratio*
	White (%)	*Black (%)*	
34–36	5.6	7.9	1.41
32–33	0.7	1.4	2
<32	0.9	2.6	2.89

Source: (Reference: 5)

often subjected to racism and disrespect from health care providers, and reports of pain or other symptoms of Black women during pregnancy are frequently disregarded (18–20). Pregnant White women do not encounter such barriers.

Many areas of the United States have been termed "maternity care deserts," because they are lacking in hospitals and birthing centers, as well as providers of obstetric care (21). In other areas, Black women give birth in hospitals that provide poorer quality health care than the hospitals where White women give birth (22).

Preterm birth has many potential serious consequences, including infant mortality; cognitive, developmental, and behavioral problems during infancy and childhood; central nervous system abnormalities; respiratory problems; gastrointestinal problems; and vision and hearing problems. Many of these problems occur because the infant does not have the 40 weeks of gestation of a full-term pregnancy, which is necessary for the brain, lungs, blood vessels, and digestive system to develop and mature. The lack of complete development of these organs and systems leaves the infant vulnerable to strokes (from undeveloped blood vessels in the brain) and other health problems. Many preterm infants spend weeks or months in neonatal intensive care units (NICUs).

The earlier a preterm infant is born, the worse the outcome. Infants born, for example, at less than 32 weeks of completed gestation (early preterm births) have worse outcomes than those born at 34–36 weeks of completed gestation (23). As shown in Table 3.4, Black infants have close to three times the risk compared to White infants of being born at less than 32 weeks of completed gestation. This means that the risk of death or other serious consequences are greater for Black than for White preterm infants.

Recent data reveal that early preterm births (<34 weeks of completed gestation) increased from 2020 to 2021, as shown in Table 3.5.

Low Birthweight

Many infants born preterm are also either low birthweight (< 2500 grams or 5.5 pounds at birth) or very low birthweight (<1500 grams or 3 pounds,

Table 3.5 Weeks of Completed Gestation for Preterm Births, by Race, United States, 2020 and 2021

Weeks of Completed Gestation (%)	*Race of Mother*		*Ratio B:W*
	White (%)	*Black (%)*	
2020			
34–36 weeks	6.90	9.54	1.38
< 34 weeks	2.21	4.82	2.18
2021			
34–36 weeks	7.18	9.8	1.36
< 34 weeks	2.31 4.94	4.94	2.14

Source: (References: 3, 4, 6)

Table 3.6 Low Birthweight Births by Race, 1970–2020

Year	*Percent Low Birthweight (< 2500 grams) by Race*		
	White	*Black*	*Ratio Black: White*
1970	6.85	13.9	2.4
1980	5.72	12.69	2.2
1990	5.7	13.25	2.3
2000	6.55	12.99	2
2005	7.16	13.59	1.9
2010	7.08	13.21	1.9
2015	6.9	13	1.88
2016	6.97	13.68	1.96
2017	7	13.89	1.98
2018	6.91	14.07	2.04
2019	6.89	14.15	2.05
2020	6.84	14.19	2.07

Source: (References: 3, 4, 6)

4 ounces at birth). Due to their birth at less than 37 weeks' gestation, preterm infants cannot gain adequate weight. As shown in Table 3.5, from 1970 to 2016, low birthweight rates fluctuated somewhat for Blacks and Whites. The ratio for low birthweight outcomes comparing Black: White infants was fairly consistent during this time, at 2.0. From 2016 through 2020, low birthweight was relatively unchanged for Whites but increased for Blacks. The ratio comparing low birthweight for Blacks: Whites from 2016 to 2020 was overall unchanged, at around 2.0.

One of the most potentially harmful birth outcomes is very low birthweight, or weight at birth of less than 1,500 grams (3 pounds, 4 ounces). As with low birthweight, from 1970 through 2020, very low birthweight fluctuated somewhat for both Whites and Blacks. The ratio comparing the percent of infants

Table 3.7 Very Low Birthweight Births by Race, 1970–2020

Year	*Percent Very Low Birthweight (< 1500 grams) by Race*		
	White	*Black*	*Ratio Black: White*
1970	0.95	2.4	2.5
1980	0.9	2.48	2.8
1990	0.95	2.92	3.1
2000	1.14	3.07	2.7
2010	1.17	2.9	2.5
2015	1.12	2.81	2.51
2016	1.07	2.95	2.8
2017	1.05	2.96	2.8
2018	1.02	2.92	2.9
2019	1.02	2.94	2.9
2020	0.99	2.86	2.9

Source: (References: 3, 4, 6)

born with very low birthweight for Blacks: Whites was overall consistent at about 3.0. The risk of death of a very low birthweight infant is very high.

It can be seen in Tables 3.3 through 3.7 that for each of the poor pregnancy outcomes presented (preterm birth, low birthweight, very low birthweight), Blacks have greater risk than Whites. This increased risk of poor pregnancy outcomes among Blacks partially explains the very high rates of infant mortality in the United States, especially for Black infants. Even Black women with higher levels of education (e.g., 16 years or more) have almost double the risk of preterm birth as their White counterparts with 16 or more years of education.

Preterm births increased substantially in the United States from 2018 to 2021 (see Table 3.3) and low birthweight births also increased from 2015 to 2020 (see Table 3.6). The increases in preterm birth and low birthweight contributed to the increases in infant mortality from 2018 to 2021, as shown in Table 3.1. The increases in preterm births and low birthweight and infant mortality can be partially attributed to the chronic stressful life conditions of pregnant women, especially Black women. Among stressful life conditions are exposure to discrimination based on race and gender (24). Thoits suggested that Black women are exposed to discrimination both due to structural and interpersonal racism and due to discrimination against women (24). Discrimination is an important type of social stressor, and chronic exposure to such stressors can increase risk of poor pregnancy outcomes through biological, psychological, or behavioral pathways (25–28).

Biological pathways include, for example, increased levels of hormones related to exposure to stressors (e.g., cortisol), which can impair the immune system. With reduced immunity, pregnant women may be more susceptible to infections (including sexually transmitted infections, bacterial vaginosis, and Group B strep), which may increase risk of preterm birth (29). Exposure to stressors may also cause an increase in blood pressure, which is associated with preeclampsia and eclampsia. These are very serious complications of pregnancy and can be life-threatening. Moreover, chronic health conditions prior to or during pregnancy, such as hypertension, can increase risk of low birthweight and preterm birth (14, 15). Hypertension and other chronic health conditions occur with greater frequency among Black women compared to White women (16).

Exposure to racial discrimination (30) and other chronic social stressors (27, 28) may also be associated with depression among pregnant women (31). Depression has been shown in prior research to increase risk of preterm birth and other poor pregnancy outcomes (11, 32, 33).

Exposure to stressful life conditions and depression are associated with behaviors that can increase the risk of preterm birth, such as smoking and use of illicit drugs (34). Depression is also associated with maternal overall health status and chronic conditions (35). Prior research has demonstrated that pregnant Black women are more likely to have prenatal depression than pregnant White women (36).

Unintended Pregnancy

Unintended pregnancies are also associated with an increased risk of preterm birth outcomes (13). Unintended pregnancies include those pregnancies that occurred sooner than desired (mistimed) or when the woman did not want to be pregnant at the time the pregnancy occurred or at any time in the future (unwanted). Pregnancies that were desired at the time they occurred or sooner are intended (13, 37). Some women report being unsure of pregnancy intendedness (13, 37). Data from the National Survey of Family Growth (NSFG) from 2006 to 2010 demonstrate that Black women have higher rates of unintended pregnancies than White women (38).

Maternal Mortality and Severe Maternal Morbidity

Another very important outcome of pregnancy is maternal mortality. The Centers for Disease Control and Prevention (CDC) defines maternal mortality as "the death of a woman during pregnancy, at delivery, or within one year of the end of the pregnancy from any cause related to or aggravated by the pregnancy." Another term used for maternal mortality is "Pregnancy-Related Death." Maternal mortality is calculated as the number of maternal deaths per 100,000 live births. Maternal mortality has increased in recent decades, from 7.2 deaths per 100,000 live births in 1987 to 17.3 per 100,000 live births in 2018 (39).

Black women have a much greater risk of maternal death compared to White women. The elevated risk of Black women for maternal mortality

Table 3.8 Maternal Mortality* for Black and White Women, United States, 1960–2016

Year	*Race of Mother*		*Ratio Black: White*
	White	*Black*	
1960	22.4	92	4.11
1970	14.4	65.5	4.55
1980	6.7	24.9	3.72
1990	5.1	21.7	4.25
2000	6.2	20.1	3.24
2005	9.1	31.7	3.48
2006	8.1	28.7	3.54
2007	7.7	23.5	3.05
2007–2008	11.5	35.6	3.1
2009–2010	12.8	41.6	3.2
2011–2012	12.4.	44.3	3.6
2013–2014	13.5	42.1	3.1
2015–2016	13.2	40.8	3.1

Source: (Reference: 41)

* Deaths per 100,000 live births.

has been termed a "Public health crisis." Black women have about three times the risk of White women of dying from pregnancy-related causes (39–47).

Table 3.8 shows maternal mortality for Black and White women from 1960 to 2016. While maternal mortality has decreased substantially during prior decades, Black women in 2015–2016 had triple the risk of death due to causes related to pregnancy and childbirth than White women.

The major causes of pregnancy-related deaths in the United States during the time period 2016–2018 include:

Cardiovascular conditions
Infection or sepsis
Cardiomyopathy
Hemorrhage
Thrombolytic pulmonary or other embolism (blood clot)
Cerebrovascular accident (stroke)
Hypertensive disorder of pregnancy
Amniotic fluid embolism
Anesthesia complications

Table 3.9 shows maternal mortality for Black and White women from 2018 to 2020. Over this time period, the ratio comparing maternal mortality of Black women to White women increased from 2.5 to 2.9.

Table 3.9 Maternal Pregnancy-Related Deaths* by Race, 2018–2020

Year	*Race of Mother*		*Ratio Black: White*
	White	*Black*	
2018	14.9	37.3	2.5
2019	17.9	44	2.46
2020	19.1	55.3	2.9

Source: (References: 40–42)

* Deaths per 100,000 live births.

Table 3.10 Maternal Mortality* by Years of Education and Race of Mother, United States, 2007–2016

Education	*Race of Mother*		*Ratio Black: White*
	Black	*White*	
< High School	45.06	25	1.8
High School	59.1	25.2	2.3
Some College	41	11.7	3.5
College Grad or More	40.2	7.8	5.2

Source: (Reference: 41)

* Deaths per 100,000 live births.

Recent research, based on data from 36 states, suggested that 34 percent of pregnancy-related deaths during the period 2017–2019 were linked to mental health issues, such as suicide and drug overdose (40). (CDC) Mental health issues were deemed the leading cause of pregnancy-related deaths during this time period. However, when the data are stratified by race, it is apparent that among Black women, the leading causes of pregnancy-related deaths were related to cardiac issues, embolism, hemorrhage, and hypertensive disorders of pregnancy (40).

Among White women, the leading cause of pregnancy-related deaths from 2017 to 2019 was mental health issues, followed by hemorrhage, cardiac issues, and infection (40).

It can be seen from Table 3.9 that from 2018 until 2020, maternal mortality rose each year for both Black and White women. For each year, maternal mortality was much higher for Black than White women. Many pregnancy-related deaths are attributed to the exposure of pregnant women, especially Black women, to chronic social stressors or stressful life conditions such as exposure to racism, job loss, poverty, or family health problems. These psychosocial factors may cause depression and health conditions such as hypertension, or inflammation, which may lead to life-threatening pregnancy complications (43).

Education does not protect Black women from death related to pregnancy or childbirth. As shown in Table 3.10, the ratio comparing maternal mortality of Black to White women is highest for women who are college graduates or have education beyond being college graduates (41, 42).

Approximately one-third of all maternal pregnancy-related deaths in the United States occur during pregnancy. Another one-third occur within one week of childbirth, and the remaining one-third occur up to one year after childbirth (40–42). Close to two-thirds of all maternal pregnancy-related deaths are considered to be preventable. One important way to prevent pregnancy-related deaths is the receipt of timely and adequate prenatal care. Black women are much less likely than White women to initiate prenatal care during the first trimester, and twice as likely to receive late or no prenatal care, as shown in Table 3.11 (19–22).

Sadly, many cases of maternal mortality could be prevented if health care providers were more responsive to symptoms of pregnancy or postpartum complications (18–20). For example, an epidemiologist with a Ph.D. from the Johns Hopkins Bloomberg School of Public Health, Dr. Shalon Irving, who worked at the CDC, died in 2017 after giving birth to a daughter. Dr. Irving experienced spikes of elevated blood pressure after having a caesarian delivery (C-section). She reported to her doctors that her legs were swollen, as was the area around her incision from the C-section delivery. She also reported headaches, blurred vision, and sudden weight gain. Her doctors dismissed her symptoms as "normal" after a C-section delivery and sent her home. She collapsed at home and died. Her education as an epidemiologist and her position at the CDC were insufficient to overcome the racism of her doctors (18, 47).

Increased risk of Black compared to White women for pregnancy-related mortality is accompanied by a greatly increased risk of severe maternal morbidity or SMM (severe illness due to complications of pregnancy) among Black women. During the period from 2016 to 2018, the risk of severe maternal morbidity among Black women was twice that of their White counterparts (226 per 10,000 births compared to 105 per 10,000 births) (48). There are approximately 50,000 to 60,000 cases of severe maternal morbidity annually in the United States (48). Many of these complications are caused due to underlying chronic health conditions of Black women, such

Table 3.11 Receipt of Prenatal Care by Race, United States, 2020

Prenatal Care (percent)	*Race*	
	White	*Black*
First Trimester	82.8	68.4
Late or No Care	4.5	9.1

Source: (Reference: 16)

Table 3.12 Fetal Death Rates per 1,000 Live Births, by Race, United States, 2018–2020

Year	*Fetal Death Rates by Race (deaths per 1,000 live births)*		
	White	*Black*	*Ratio Black: White*
2018	4.89	10.64	2.18
2019	4.71	10.41	2.21
2020	4.73	10.34	2.19

Source: (Reference: 49)

as hypertension or obesity. Black women have greater risk of these chronic health conditions than White women (16).

Fetal Death

Another important deleterious outcome of pregnancy is fetal death. Fetal death is the death of the fetus in utero at any time during the pregnancy (49). Fetal deaths after 20 weeks of gestation are termed "stillbirths." The major causes of fetal deaths are:

Disorders of the placenta, cord, or membranes;
Maternal pregnancy complications;
Congenital malformations;
Maternal health conditions not related to the pregnancy.

As shown in Table 3.12, Black women have over twice the risk of their White counterparts of Fetal Death.

Summary

Black women, compared to White women, have increased risk for each measure of poor maternal, pregnancy, and infant health outcomes. For several measures, such as maternal mortality and infant mortality, there have been increases in recent years. In order to reduce infant mortality, maternal mortality, preterm birth, low birthweight, fetal deaths, and severe maternal morbidity in the United States, especially among Black women, it will be necessary to better understand the relationship between the social environment with maternal health and pregnancy outcomes. Demonstration projects of providing support to pregnant women and new mothers have shown that social support can improve outcomes of pregnancy for mothers and infants (50, 51). These efforts will be helped by increased investment in family supports.

Prior research has also demonstrated that health-enhancing resources, such as social support, can mitigate the impact of exposure to social stressors, thereby improving pregnancy outcomes (52, 53). The Surgeon General of the United States recently called attention to the significant negative health impact of social isolation and loneliness (54).

With new knowledge about Social Determinants of Health, and increased investment in health-enhancing resources, it will be possible to intervene with women with increased risk of poor maternal, pregnancy, and infant health outcomes to improve the social environment, and improve the maternal, pregnancy, and infant health outcomes of Black women. Improving the social environment includes both reducing exposure to social stressors (e.g., racism, poverty, housing, work, and neighborhood problems, problems with the legal system, lack of access to health care) (30, 55, 56), and providing health-enhancing resources such as food security, neighborhood family support centers, or home visitation programs.

Underlying the poor maternal, pregnancy, and infant health outcomes in the United States for centuries is racial discrimination (55–57). The great public health challenge of our time (58) is to find the political will as a nation to confront and eliminate racism (57). This is the only road to achieve maternal, pregnancy, and infant health outcomes equal to those of other high-income countries (59). This is an issue not only of health equity but of social justice.

References

1 *America's Health Rankings, Health of Women and Children*. Minnetonka, MN: United Health Foundation, 2022.

2 *March of Dimes, Peristats- March of Dimes Report Card, Perinatal Data Center*. Arlington, VA: March of Dimes, 2022.

3 Ely M, Driscoll AK. Infant mortality in the United States, 2019: data from the period linked birth/infant death file. *National Vital Statistics Reports, 70 (14)*. Hyattsville, MD: National Center for Health Statistics, 2021.

4 Ely DM, Driscoll AK. Infant mortality in the United States, 2018: data from the period linked Birth/Infant death file. *National Vital Statistics Reports, 69 (7)*. Hyattsville, MD: National Center for Health Statistics, 2020.

5 *Health United States 2019*. Hyattsville, MD: National Center for Health Statistics, 2020.

6 *Health United States 2020–2021*. Hyattsville, MD: National Center for Health Statistics, 2022.

7 Cassidy-Wu L, Wan V, Spangler J. The correlation between food insecurity and infant mortality in North Carolina. *Public Health Nutr* 2022; 25: 1038–1044.

8 Behrman RE, Butler AS (eds). *Preterm Birth: Causes, Consequences and Prevention*. Washington, DC: Institute of Medicine, National Academies Press, 2007.

9 Hamilton BE, Martin JA, Osterman MSK. Births: provisional data for 2021. *Vital Statistics Rapid Release No. 20*. Hyattsville, MD: National Center for Health Statistics, May 2022.

10 Dole N, Savitz DA, Hertz-Picciotto I, et al. Maternal stress and preterm birth. *Am J Epidemiol* 2003; 157: 14–24.

11 Orr ST, James SA, Blackmore-Prince C. Maternal prenatal depressive symptoms and spontaneous preterm birth among African Ameri can women in Baltimore, MD. *Am J Epidemiol* 2002; 156: 797–802.
12 Orr ST, Reiter JP, Blazer DG, James SA. Pregnancy-related anxiety and spontaneous preterm birth in Baltimore, MD. *Psychosom Med* 2007; 69: 566–570.
13 Orr ST, Miller CA, James SA, Babones S. Unintended pregnancy and preterm birth. *Paediatr Perinat Epidemiol* 2000; 14: 309–313.
14 Orr ST, Reiter JP, James SA, Orr CA. Maternal health prior to pregnancy and preterm birth among urban low income Black women in Baltimore: the Baltimore Preterm Birth Study. *Ethn Dis* 2011; 22: 85–89.
15 Orr ST, Blackmore-Prince C, James SA, et al. Race, clinical factors, and pregnancy outcome in a low-income urban setting. *Ethn Dis* 2000; 10: 411–417.
16 Office of Minority Health. *Policy and Data, Profiles, Black/African American Health*. Washington, DC: United States Department of Health and Human Services, 2023.
17 Fleishman R. You can do everything right and still have a preterm birth. *Time*, October 28, 2022.
18 Purnell TS, Irving W, Irving S, et al. Honoring Dr. Shalom Irving: a champion for health equity. *Health Aff* 2022; 41: 304–308.
19 Cotton TM. I was pregnant and in crisis and all the doctors saw was an incompetent Black woman. *Time*, January 5, 2019.
20 Ward S, Mazul M, Ngui EM, et al. "You learn to go last:" perceptions of prenatal care experiences among African-American women with limited incomes. *Mater Child Health J* 2013; 17: 1753–1759.
21 *Nowhere to Go: Maternity Care Deserts Across the United States*. Arlington, VA: March of Dimes, 2022.
22 Sutton MY, Anachebe NF, Lee R, Skanes S. Racial and ethnic disparities in reproductive health services and outcomes, 2020. *Obstet Gynecol* 2021; 137: 225–233.
23 Osterman M, Hamilton B, Martin J, et al. Births: final data for 2020. *National Vital Statistics Reports 70 (17)*. Hyattsville, MD: National Center for Health Statistics, 2022.
24 Thoits P. Race and gender stress and health: major findings and policy implications. *J Health Soc Behav* 2010; 51 (Suppl): S41–S53.
25 Williams DR, Lawrence JA, Davis BA, Vu C. Understanding how discrimination can affect health. *Health Serv Res* 2019; 54: 1374–1388.
26 Bower K, Geller RJ, Perrin NA, Alhusen J. Experiences of racism and preterm birth: findings from a Pregnancy Risk Assessment Monitoring System, 2004 through 2018. *Health Issues* 2018; 28: 495–501.
27 Orr ST, James SA, Casper R. Psychosocial stressors and low birthweight: development of a questionnaire. *J Dev Behav Pediatr* 1992; 13: 343–347.
28 Orr ST, James SA, Miller CA, et al. Psychosocial stressors and low birthweight in an urban population. *Am J Prev Med* 1996; 12: 459–466.
29 Goldenberg RL, Hauth JC, Andrews WW. Intrauterine infection and preterm delivery. *NEJM* 2000; 342: 1500–1507.
30 Bailey ZD, Krieger N, Agenor M, et al. Structural racism and health inequities in the USA: evidence and interventions. *Lancet* 2017; 40: 105–125.
31 Orr ST, James SA, Burns BJ, Thompson B. Chronic stressors and maternal depression: implications for prevention. *Am J Public Health* 1989; 10: 287–289.

32 Hoffman S, Hatch MC. Depressive symptomatology during pregnancy: evidence for an association with decreased fetal growth in pregnancies of lower social class women. *Health Psychol* 2000; 19: 535–543.
33 Staneeva A, Bogossin F, Pritchard M, Wittkowski A. The effects of maternal depression, anxiety and perceived stress during pregnancy on preterm birth: a systematic review. *Womens Birth* 2015; 28: 179–193.
34 Orr ST, Newton ER, Tarwater PM, Weismiller D. Factors associated with prenatal smoking among Black women in eastern North Carolina. *Maternal Child Health J* 2005; 9: 245–252.
35 Orr ST, Blazer DG, James SA, Reiter J. Depressive symptoms and indicators of maternal health status during pregnancy. *J Womens Health* 2007; 16: 535–542.
36 Orr ST, Blazer DG, James SA. Racial disparities in elevated prenatal depressive symptoms among Black and White women in eastern North Carolina. *Ann Epidemiol* 2006; 16: 463–468.
37 Brown S, Eisenberg L. *The Best Intentions: Unintended Pregnancy and the Well-being of Children and Families*. Washington, DC: National Academies Press, 1995.
38 Mosher WD, Jones J, Abma JC. Intended and unintended births in the United States 1982–2010. *National Vital Statistics Reports 55*. Hyattsville, MD: National Center for Health Statistics, July 2012.
39 Declerq E, Zephyrin L. *Maternal Mortality in the United States: A Primer*. New York: Commonwealth Fund, December 2020.
40 Hoyert DL. *Maternal Mortality Rates in the United States, 2020*. Hyattsville, MD: National Center for Health Statistics, Health e-stats, 2022.
41 Petersen EE, Davis NL, Goodman D, et.al. Racial/ethnic disparities in pregnancy-related deaths – United States, 2007–2016. *Morb Mortal Wkly Rep* 2019; 68 (35): 762–765.
42 Petersen EE, Davis N, Goodman D, et al. Pregnancy-related deaths, United States, 2011–2015, and strategies for prevention, 17 states, 2013–2017. *Morb Mortal Wkly Rep*. 2019; 68 (18): 423–429.
43 Gunja MZ, Gums ED, Williams RD. *The U.S. Maternal Mortality Crisis Continues to Worsen: An International Comparison*. New York: Commonwealth Fund, 2022.
44 Lu MC. Reducing maternal mortality in the United States. *JAMA* 2018; 320: 1237–1238.
45 *America Already Had a Maternal Mortality Crisis. It's Getting Even Worse*. Washington, DC: Century Foundation, October 12, 2022.
46 *America's Maternal Mortality Crisis Is Worsening*. Washington, DC: Century Foundation, April 4, 2023.
47 Martin N, Montagne R. Nothing protects Black women from dying in pregnancy and childbirth. *Pro Publica*, December 7, 2017.
48 Declerq E, Zephyrin L. *Severe Maternal Morbidity in the United States: A Primer*. New York: Commonwealth Fund, October 2021.
49 Gregory ECW, Valenzuela CP, Hoyer DL. Fetal mortality: United States, 2020. *Natl Vital Stat Syst* 2022; 71 (4).
50 Olds DL. Prenatal and infancy home visiting by nurses: from randomized trials to community replications. *Prev Sci* 2002; 3: 153–172.
51 Olds D, Sadler L, Kitzman H. Programs for parents of infants and toddlers: recent evidence from randomized trials. *J Child Psychol Psychiatr* 2017; 48: 355–391.

52 Orr ST. Social support and pregnancy outcome: a review of the literature. *Clin Obstet Gynecol* 2004; 47: 842–855.
53 Nuckolls KB, Kaplan B, Cassel JC. Psychosocial assets, life crises, and the prognosis of pregnancy. *Am J Epidemiol* 1972; 95: 431–441.
54 *Our Epidemic of Loneliness and Isolation: The US Surgeon General's Advisory on the Healing Effects of Social Connection and Community*. Washington, DC: United States Department of Health and Human Services, 2023.
55 Rosenberg L, Palmer JR, Wise LA, et al. Perceptions of racial discrimination and the risk of preterm birth. *Epidemiol* 2002; 13: 646–652.
56 Bailey ZD, Feldman JA, Bassett MF. How structural racism works- racial policies as a root cause of US racial health inequities. *NEJM* 2021; 384: 768–773.
57 James SA. Confronting the moral economy of US racial/ethnic health disparities. *Am J Public Health* 2003; 93: 189.
58 Williams DR, Purdue-Vaughns V. Needed interventions to reduce racial/ethnic disparities in health. *J Health Polit Policy Law* 2016; 41: 627–651.
59 Weintraub K. Americans' life expectancy continues to fall, erasing health gains of the last quarter century. *USA Today*, December 22, 2022.

4 The COVID-19 Pandemic and Black Women

Inequities in Hospitalization and Death From COVID-19 Among Young Black Women

In early 2020, as the pandemic of COVID-19 swept across the world, causing millions of hospitalizations and deaths, it became apparent that in the United States, Blacks were disproportionately affected by this virus. While initially, data for deaths and hospitalizations from COVID-19 by race and gender were difficult to obtain for the United States, it became clear that Blacks were more likely than Whites to be hospitalized and to die from this severe viral illness (1–11). An awakening to health inequities and injustice accompanied the spread of COVID-19, with the recognition of the increased risk of Blacks compared to Whites for death and hospitalization from COVID-19. Blacks clearly bore a disproportionate burden of COVID-19, compared to Whites (1–11).

According to one author (2), the COVID-19 pandemic exploited systems that were already failing in the United States, such as overcrowded prisons, understaffed nursing homes, and an underfunded public health system. These failing systems led to the United States having 16 percent of the world's deaths from COVID-19, despite having only 4 percent of the world's population (2).

Overall, the COVID-19 pandemic caused a much greater loss of life in the United States than in other high-resource nations around the world (12–15). Despite spending more per capita on health care than other wealthy nations, the outcomes for infection with COVID-19 in the United States were worse than those of other high-resource nations.

The impact of COVID-19 infection in the United States is reflected in data about changes in life expectancy at birth and mortality from 2019 to 2020. Life expectancy at birth declined for both Black and White women in the United States from 2019 to 2020, and the difference in life expectancy at birth between Black and White women increased (16, 17). Moreover, age-adjusted all-cause mortality increased from 2019 to 2020 among both Black and White women. The increase was much greater for Black women (+24.9 percent) than for White women (+12.1 percent), and the ratio comparing age-adjusted all-cause mortality for Black: White women increased from 2019

DOI:10.4324/9781032663807-4

to 2020 (18). These data, shown in Chapter 2 of this book, demonstrate the much greater impact of COVID-19 upon mortality among Black women compared to White women. Black women in the United States have greater mortality from COVID-19 than any other group except Black men (18).

The same groups that bore a disproportionate burden of COVID-19 in the United States also suffer from a disproportionate burden of many other diseases. As discussed in other chapters in this book, young Black women have an increased risk of mortality, compared to young White women, from various leading causes of death, including certain cancers, cardiovascular disease, stroke, diabetes, and HIV/AIDS (19). These underlying conditions make Black women more likely to become severely ill or to die from COVID-19 compared to White women. The increased risk of Black women, compared to White women, of underlying chronic health conditions, such as cardiovascular disease and cancer, can be attributed to the exposure of Black women to high levels of social stressors, such as racial discrimination, poverty, and job and neighborhood-related stressful conditions (20–24).

Much of the strategy for controlling the pandemic has been focused upon immunizations and medical therapeutics (e.g., antiretroviral medications), rather than a public health approach, which is focused upon prevention (2). The focus in the United States upon the use of clinical (biomedical) tools cannot be effective if the populations at greatest risk of death, such as Blacks, do not have adequate access to these tools. Many Black women cannot miss work to make and keep appointments for receipt of immunizations. There needs to be a change in focus, to address the social conditions that foster racial inequities in health, such as exposure to chronic, ongoing stressors (such as racial discrimination, economic, employment, and housing instability), lack of health insurance, or the racism that makes access to preventive health care among young Black women so difficult (25).

Overall, the percentage of the population of the United States that is Black (approximately 12 percent) is far lower than the percentage of deaths and hospitalizations from COVID-19 among Blacks. For example, in Chicago, about one-third of the population is Black, but Blacks comprised 72 percent of deaths from COVID-19 in 2020 (4). Similarly, in Michigan, Blacks comprise 14 percent of the population, but 40 percent of all deaths from COVID-19 in 2020 (4). In New Orleans, Blacks are less than one-third of the population, but about 40 percent of deaths from COVID-19 in 2021 (4).

One study showed that those counties in the United States with a higher proportion of Blacks in the population (13 percent or more) had greater mortality from COVID-19 compared to those counties with lower percentages of Blacks in the population (less than 13 percent) (5).

Social Determinants of Health and COVID-19

Blacks are more likely to become seriously ill or die from COVID-19 for several potential reasons. First, they are subjected to various types of ongoing, chronic social stressors, such as racism, neighborhood crime, and poverty. Exposure to such chronic social stressors can weaken the immune system, making Blacks more susceptible to severe illness and death. In addition, Blacks are more likely than Whites to have various chronic underlying health conditions, such as hypertension, heart disease, and diabetes. The presence of these chronic health conditions makes them more vulnerable to severe illness and death from COVID-19.

In a recent talk titled "Pandemic Preparedness and Response: Lessons Learned From COVID-19," renowned NIH (National Institutes of Health) infectious disease scientist Dr. Anthony Fauci discussed the magnitude of the racial disparities in mortality from COVID-19. Dr. Fauci emphasized the role of Social Determinants of Health in the excess risk of mortality from COVID-19 in the United States among Blacks compared to Whites. He ascribed the increased risk among Blacks of severe illness and death to underlying socially determined chronic conditions, poverty, and crowded housing conditions that did not allow distancing within the household (25).

Racial Disparities in Treatment for COVID-19

In a recently published paper, it was reported that Blacks infected with COVID-19 were less likely to be treated with newer antiviral medications or monoclonal antibodies than Whites with COVID-19 (26). For example, Black patients were 35 percent less likely to be treated with Paxlovid than White patients with COVID-19 infection (26). The sample for this study included approximately 700,000 patients who sought medical care for COVID-19. About 14 percent of the sample consisted of Black patients, and 68 percent were White, similar to the population of the United States. The patients were 20 years of age and older, seen at 30 treatment sites from January through July 2022 (26).

Deaths From COVID-19 Among Young Black Women and Impact on Families

In 2020, COVID-19 became the third-leading cause of death among Black and White women overall (18). However, this is somewhat misleading, due to the differences observed in the ten leading causes of death by age group. Among women aged 15–24 years, COVID-19 was the seventh-leading cause of death for both Black and White women in 2020. For women aged 25–34 years, among White women, COVID-19 was the seventh-leading cause of death in 2020, but among Black women in this age group, COVID-19 was the fifth-leading cause of death. For women aged 35–44 years, COVID-19 was the sixth-leading cause of death for White women, but the fourth-leading cause of death for Black women in 2020. These differences in mortality suggest more severe illnesses and death among Black women compared to White women in 2020.

The death of a woman in the "prime of life" (ages 20–45 years), when she is a mother, wife, daughter, sister, friend, neighbor, worker, church member, and community volunteer is a tragic loss, creating a void in Black families and communities. Children left without a mother, their primary caregiver, are likely to suffer the effects of this loss for a lifetime (27). A child's loss of their primary caregiver (usually the mother) due to death from COVID-19 has been termed a "hidden pandemic" (27).

In the United States, over 142,000 children suffered the loss of their primary caregiver (usually their mother, but the primary caregiver could be a grandparent or other family member) due to the COVID-19 pandemic (27). These losses disproportionately impacted Black children, since the risk of dying from COVID-19 among Blacks was over twice that of Whites (27). The loss of a primary caregiver due to COVID-19 infection occurred to 1 in 310 Black children and 1 in 753 White children (27). In other words, Black children were over twice as likely as White children to suffer the loss of their primary caregiver due to COVID-19. Therefore, proportionately more Black than White children will suffer from the long-term mental health and other consequences of losing the primary caregiver.

Some children even suffered the loss of a primary caregiver twice. For example, if their mother died (from either COVID-19 infection or other causes prior to or during the pandemic), and the grandmother became the primary caregiver, and then she died as well, the child would suffer the loss of their primary caregiver twice. These Adverse Childhood Experiences (orphanhood) are associated with subsequent mental health problems, increased substance use, increased suicide, and decreased years of completed schooling (27). Black children may suffer the mental health and other consequences of the loss of a parent for decades.

Long COVID Among Young Black Women

The phenomenon known as "long COVID" (also known as post-COVID conditions) may affect Black women after infection with COVID-19. Little is known or understood about "long COVID," but it is apparent that many people infected with COVID-19 may experience symptoms for weeks, months, or longer after the initial illness (28, 29). These symptoms may include fatigue, fever, muscle or joint pain, rash, shortness of breath, and cough. Other symptoms may include chest pain and heart palpitations, "brain fog," headache, sleep problems, lightheadedness, and the sensation of "pins and needles." Mental health symptoms may occur as well, including depression and anxiety. New health conditions may also arise among Black women after COVID-19 infection, such as diabetes, hypertension, or heart disease.

These symptoms may have a negative impact on the ability of Black women to function as workers, parents, wives, daughters, etc., after illness with COVID-19. Families may face severe economic difficulties, or poverty, if the mother cannot work due to post-COVID conditions. Even prior to the pandemic, Black women were more likely than White women to be poor (30). Black women often report difficulties affording basic necessities such as rent and utilities (31). Inability to work due to post-COVID conditions will exacerbate economic problems for Black women.

The risk of developing long COVID is increased among those who have more severe illness with COVID-19, are unvaccinated, or have underlying health conditions such as diabetes or hypertension. Black women are more likely than White women to have more severe illness due to COVID-19 infection, to be unvaccinated (32), and to have underlying health conditions such as diabetes, which place them at increased risk of developing long COVID (19). The consequences of long COVID among young Black women may include the inability to work, help other family members, and function as parents.

Summary

COVID-19 has disproportionately affected Black compared to White women in the United States. The only group in the population with greater mortality from COVID-19, compared to Black women, was Black men (18). The many deleterious effects of COVID-19 upon Black women in the prime of life and their families include the potential loss of the mother, economic hardship, and health problems due to long COVID (chronic physical and mental health conditions).

The pandemic shined a light on the many inequities and injustices that affect the health of Black women. The shocking events that occurred due to racial discrimination during the pandemic, including the killing of George Floyd and Breonna Taylor by police, drew increased attention to the widespread racism in the United States (7). This increased the exposure to stressors in the social environment by young Black women and added to insecurity and loss of predictability and hope.

Racial discrimination is a major social stressor to which Black women are exposed, beginning at young ages (20–23). Racism impacts essentially all aspects of the lives of young Black women, from health to economic status, to job insecurity to housing conditions (21–23).

In order to truly improve the health of young Black women, it will be necessary to confront the widespread racism in the United States and to focus on equity, diversity, and inclusiveness in schools, communities, workplaces, and health care settings (7, 20, 33–38). Racism by the justice system and police must also be addressed. Only by reducing exposure to social stressors will it be possible to achieve health equity for Black women.

The pandemic of COVID-19 highlighted the health inequities in the United States, forcing attention to be paid to the unjust circumstances in the social environment that allowed COVID-19 to take such a disproportionate toll on Black women (20–23). As the United States moves forward to address inequities in health, it will be necessary to closely examine, understand, and reduce these inequities that prevent young Black women from achieving optimal health.

In order to reduce the toll of COVID-19 on young Black women, it will be necessary to address issues which include disease prevention (the public health approach), inequality, and racism, and to prioritize the needs of the most vulnerable groups (20, 33–38). It was noted by Carratala and Maxwell that "[a]lleviating health disparities will require deliberate and sustained effort to address social determinants of health, such as poverty, segregation, environmental degradation, and racial discrimination" (38). It will also be necessary not only to reduce those aspects of the social environment that negatively impact health of young Black women but to increase the "health enhancing" factors that can mitigate the impact of exposure to stressors (39, 40).

Finally, there is a need in the United States to develop the political will to eliminate racial discrimination and other aspects of the Social Determinants of Health that threaten the health of young Black women (17, 20, 37). Social and economic policies need to be developed that will improve the lives and life circumstances of young Black women, thereby improving their health, so that equity in health can be achieved (41).

References

1 Yong E. How the pandemic will end. *Atlantic*, March 25, 2020
2 Yong E. How the pandemic defeated America. *Atlantic*, September 2020.
3 Yong E. The pandemic's legacy is already clear. *Atlantic*, September 20, 2022.
4 Grace D, Johnson C, Reid T. Racial inequalities and COVID-19. *Greenlining*, 2020.
5 Millett GA, Jones MA, Sullivan PS, et al. Assessing differential impacts of COVID-19 on black communities. *Ann Epidemiol* 2020; 47: 37–44.
6 Luck AN, Preston SH, Alo IT, Stokes AC. The unequal burden of the COVID-19 pandemic: capturing racial/ethnic disparities in United States cause-specific mortality. *SSM Popul Health* 2022; 17: 101012.
7 Galea S, Abdella SM. COVID-19 pandemic, unemployment, and civil unrest: underlying deep racial and socioeconomic divides. *JAMA* 2020; 324: 227–228.
8 Johnson A, Buford T. Early data shows African Americans have contracted and died of Coronavirus at an alarming rate. *Pro Publica*, April 3, 2020.
9 Ray R. *Why Are Blacks Dying at Higher Rates from COVID-19?* Washington, DC: Brookings Inst, April 9, 2020.
10 *COVID-19 Response Health Equity Strategy: Accelerating Progress Towards Reducing COVID-19 Disparities and Achieving Health Equity*. Atlanta: Center for Disease Control and Prevention, 2022.
11 Andrasfey T, Goldman N. Reductions in 2020 United States life expectancy due to COVID-19 and the disproportionate impact in the Black and Latino populations. *Proc Natl Acad Sci* 2021; 118: e2014746118.
12 Woolf SH, Chapman DA, Sabo RT, Zimmerman EB. Excess deaths from COVID-19 and other causes in the United States, March 1, 2020 to January 2, 2021. *JAMA* 2022; 325: 1786–1789.
13 Mueller B, Lutz E. United States has far higher COVID death rate than other wealthy countries. *New York Times*, February 1, 2022.
14 Woolf SH. Effect of the COVID-19 pandemic in 2020 on life expectancy across populations in the USA. *BMJ* 2021; 373: n1343.

15 Barbieri M. Editorial: COVID-19 and the growing disadvantage in United States life expectancy. *BMJ* 2021; 373: n1530.
16 Arias E, Tejada-Vera B, Ahmad F, Kochanek KD. Provisional life expectancy estimates for 2020. *Vital Statistics Rapid Release No. 15*. Hyattsville, MD: National Center for Health Statistics, July 2021.
17 Weintraub K. Americans' life expectancy continues to fall, erasing health gains of the last quarter century. *USA Today*, December 22, 2022.
18 Murphy SL, Kochanek KD, Xu J, Arias E. Mortality in the United States, 2020. *Data Brief 427*. Hyattsville, MD: National Center for Health Statistics, December 2021.
19 Office of Minority Health. *Policy and Data: Black/African American Profile*. Washington, DC: United States Department of Health and Human Services, 2023.
20 James SA. Confronting the moral economy of US racial/ethnic health disparities. *Am J Public Health* 2003; 93: 189.
21 Williams DR, Lawrence JA, Davis BA, Vu C. Understanding how discrimination can affect health. *Health Serv Res* 2019; 54 (Suppl 2): 1374–1388.
22 Williams DR, Lawrence JA, Davis BA. Racism and health: evidence and needed research. *Ann Rev Public Health* 2019; 40: 15–125.
23 Bailey ZD, Feldman JM, Bassett MT. How structural racism works – racist policies as a root cause of US racial health inequities. *NEJM* 2021; 384: 768–773.
24 Frye J. *On the Frontlines at Work and at Home: The Disproportionate Effects of the Coronavirus Pandemic on Women of Color*. Washington, DC: Center for American Progress, April 23, 2020.
25 Fauci A. *Pandemic Preparedness and Response: Lessons from COVID-19. Department of Medicine Grand Rounds*. Ralph Nachman, MD: Visiting Professorship. Weill Cornell Medicine, March 29, 2023.
26 Boehner TK, Koumans EH, Skillen EL, et al. Racial and ethnic disparities in outpatient treatment of COVID-19 – United States, June–July 2022. *Morb Mortal Wkly Rep* 2022; 71 (43): 1359–1365.
27 Hillis SD, Bienkinsop A, Villeveces A, et al. COVID-19-associated orphanhood and caregiver deaths in the United States. *Pediatrics* 2021; 148: e2021053760.ss
28 Burns A. *Will Long COVID Exacerbate Existing Disparities in Health and Employment?* San Francisco: Kaiser Family Foundation, September 23, 2022.
29 Berger Z, deJesus VA, Greenhalgh T. Long COVID and health inequities: the role of primary care. *Milbank Q* 2021; 99: 519–541.
30 Bleiweis R, Boesch D, Gaines AC. *The Basic Facts about Women and Poverty*. Washington, DC: Center for American Progress, August 3, 2020.
31 Orr ST, James SA, Casper R. Psychosocial stressors and low birthweight: development of a questionnaire. *J Dev Behav Pediatr* 1992; 13: 343–347.
32 Ndugga N, Hill L, Jones ATS, Haldar S. *Latest Data on COVID-19 Vaccination by Race/Ethnicity*. San Francisco: Kaiser Family Foundation, July 14, 2022.
33 Satcher D, Higginbotham EJ. The public health approach to eliminating disparities in health. *Am J Public Health* 2008; 98 (Suppl): S8–S11.
34 Williams DR, Purdue-Vaughns V. Needed interventions to reduce racial/ethnic disparities in health. *J Health Polit Policy Law* 2016; 41: 627–651.
35 Woolf SH. *Social and Economic Policies Can Help to Reverse Americans' Declining Health*. Washington, DC: Center for American Progress, September 2021.

36 Thornton R, Glover C, Cene C, et al. Evaluating strategies for reducing health disparities by addressing the social determinants of health. *Health Aff* 2016; 35: 1416–1423.
37 Miller CA. Societal change and public health: a rediscovery. *Am J Public Health* 1976; 66: 54–60.
38 Carratala S, Maxwell C. *Health Disparities by Race and Ethnicity*. Washington, DC: Center for American Progress, May 7, 2020.
39 Orr ST. Social support and pregnancy outcome: a review of the literature. *Clin Obstet Gynecol* 2004; 47: 842–855.
40 Thoits PA. Mechanisms linking social ties and support to physical and mental health. *J Health Soc Behav* 2011; 52: 145–161.
41 Woolf SH. Social policy as health policy. *JAMA* 2009; 301: 1166–1169.

5 Cardiovascular Disease and Cerebrovascular Disease

Introduction

Cardiovascular (heart) disease and cerebrovascular disease (stroke) are among the leading causes of death for Black and White women in the United States. They are combined into one chapter, because overall, the same factors (e.g., hypertension) increase risk for mortality and morbidity for both conditions.

Diseases of the Heart

Cardiovascular disease is the leading cause of death for both Black and White women of all ages in the United States. However, this statement is somewhat misleading. For younger women, there are other causes of death that occur with greater frequency than heart disease. The greatest mortality from cardiovascular disease is among older women. For younger women (20–44 years of age), cardiovascular disease is among the top ten causes of death but is not the leading cause of death (1–3). For Black women, cardiovascular disease was the third-leading cause of death for women aged 20–44 years in 2018 (2, 4). For White women, cardiovascular disease was the fourth-leading cause of death among women aged 20–44 years in 2018 (2, 4).

Table 5.1 shows the age-adjusted mortality rates per 100,000 population for diseases of the heart among Black and White women from 1950 to 2019. It can be seen from this table that since 1950, the age-adjusted mortality from cardiovascular disease has decreased for both Black and White women. However, from 1950 until 2019, Black women had higher rates of mortality from diseases of the heart than White women. Moreover, the ratio comparing mortality from diseases of the heart for Black: White women increased from 1950 to 2019, from 1.1 in 1950 to 1.3 from 1990 until 2019.

As noted previously, among women in younger age groups, cardiovascular disease is not the leading cause of death for Black or White women, despite being the leading cause of death among both groups overall (i.e., for all ages) (9). In 2019, among women aged 15–19 and 20–24 years, cardiovascular

DOI: 10.4324/9781032663807-5

Table 5.1 Age-Adjusted Mortality for Cardiovascular Disease per 100,000 Population Among Women, by Race, United States, 1950–2019

Year	*Race*		
	White Females	*Black Females*	*Ratio Black: White*
1950	479.2	538.9	1.12
1960	441.7	488.9	1.11
1970	376.7	435.6	1.16
1980	315.9	378.6	1.2
1990	250.9	327.5	1.31
2000	205.6	277.6	1.35
2013	132	172.1	1.3
2015	130	167.7	1.3
2019	130.7	168.6	1.3

Source: (References: 2–8)

Table 5.2 Ratios Comparing Age-Adjusted Mortality Rates for Diseases of the Heart for Black: White Women by Age Group, 2019

Age Group (years)	*Ratio of Mortality Rates Comparing Black: White Women*
15–19	2.45
20–24	2.68
25–34	2.41
35–44	2.58

Source: (References: 3, 4, 6, 8)

disease was the fourth-leading cause of death for Black women and the fifth-leading cause of death for White women. Among women aged 25–34 years, in 2019 cardiovascular disease was the second-leading cause of death for Black women and the fourth-leading cause of death for White women. Finally, in 2019, among women aged 35–44 years, heart disease was the second-leading cause of death among Black women and the third-leading cause of death among White women. For each of these age groups, as shown in Table 5.2, Black women had much higher age-adjusted mortality per 100,000 population than White women (3–8).

There are several different types of cardiovascular disease. These include:

Coronary artery disease: This is the most common type of heart disease. It is caused by arteriosclerosis, narrowing and hardening of the coronary arteries.

Congestive heart failure: This type of heart disease is caused by hypertension and obesity. With congestive heart failure, the heart muscle cannot pump adequately.

Other types of diseases of the heart include heart arrhythmia (abnormal rhythm of the heartbeat); heart valve disease; rheumatic heart disease; congenital heart disease; diseases of the heart muscle (associated with diabetes, hypertension, and obesity); and myocardial infarction (termed "heart attack," which occurs when a coronary artery is blocked by a blood clot).

Cerebrovascular Disease (Stroke)

As shown in Table 5.3, the age-adjusted mortality per 100,000 population from stroke decreased substantially from 1950 to 2019. However, the ratio comparing Black: White women for stroke mortality was the same in 1950 as in 2019. The ratio of stroke mortality for Black: White women (comparing age-adjusted mortality per 100,000 population) was 1.4 in 1950 and 1.38 in 2019. From 2000 until 2014, the ratio declined to 1.3 but increased in 2019 (3–8).

As with cardiovascular disease, mortality from cerebrovascular disease varies by age among Black and White women (3, 9). In 2019, for both Black and White women aged 15–19 and 20–24, stroke was not among the ten leading causes of death. Among women aged 25–34, the age-adjusted mortality per 100,000 population for Black women was 2.3, and for White women, it was 1.1 (ratio Black: White women = 2.09). In 2019, among Black women aged 35–44, the age-adjusted mortality per 100,000 population was 5.4, while for White women in this age group, the mortality from stroke was 3.2 (ratio Black: White women = 1.69) (3, 4, 6, 8).

At all ages, Black women have greater mortality from stroke than their White counterparts. Table 5.4 shows the ratio for mortality from stroke comparing Black: White women for various age groups. As shown in this table, for each age group, Black women had greater mortality rates (age-adjusted per 100,000 population) than their White counterparts.

Table 5.3 Age-Adjusted Mortality for Cerebrovascular Disease per 100,000 Population Among Women, by Race, United States, 1950–2019

Year	*Race*		
	White	*Black*	*Ratio Black: White*
1950	169.7	238.4	1.4
1960	165	232.5	1.41
1970	135.5	189.3	1.4
1980	89	119.6	1.34
1990	60.3	84	1.39
2000	57.3	76.2	1.33
2014	34.7	45.2	1.3
2019	35.6	48	1.3

Source: (References: 4, 6, 8)

Table 5.4 Ratios Comparing Age-Adjusted Mortality Rates for Stroke for Black: White Women, by Age Group, 2019

Age Group (years)	*Ratio of Mortality Rates Comparing Black: White Women*
15–19	n/a
20–24	n/a
25–34	2.2
35–44	2.4

Source: (References: 3, 4, 6, 8)

There are two major types of cerebrovascular disease. One is Ischemic Stroke. In this type of stroke, fatty deposits inside blood vessels create obstructions in the cerebral blood vessels. These blockages hinder circulation of blood to and within the brain. Ischemic Strokes account for 87 percent of all strokes.

The other major type of stroke is Hemorrhagic Stroke, in which a weakened blood vessel within the brain ruptures, and the pressure of the blood within the tissues of the brain causes damage to the brain. Uncontrolled hypertension causes most Hemorrhagic Strokes.

Health Factors and Risk of Cardiovascular Disease and Stroke

Several underlying health conditions increase the risk of morbidity and mortality from cardiovascular disease and stroke. One such factor is hypertension. In 2018, among Black women aged 18 years or older, 56.7 percent reported that they had hypertension, compared to 36.7 percent of White women. (These data are self-reported and age-adjusted.) The ratio comparing self-reported hypertension in 2018 among Black: White women was 1.5 (10).

Another underlying health condition that increases risk of cardiovascular disease and stroke is diabetes mellitus. During the period 2017–2018, among women aged 18 and older, the age-adjusted percentage with diabetes among Black women was 12.0 percent, compared to 6.6 percent of White women. The ratio comparing Black: White women was 1.8 (10).

In 2018, the age-adjusted mortality from diabetes per 100,000 population was 33.1 for Black women and 14.3 for White women (ratio Black: White women = 2.3) (10, 11).

Overweight (body mass index or BMI of 25 or greater) and obesity (BMI of 30 or greater) also increase the risk of heart disease and stroke. Approximately four of five Black women are overweight or obese. Black women have the highest rates of overweight or obesity of any population group (10).

During the period from 2013 to 2016, among adults aged 20 years or older, the prevalence of overweight and obesity (BMI of 25 or greater) was

80.6 percent for Black women. The prevalence of overweight or obesity in 2013–2016 was 64.8 percent for White women. The ratio comparing Black: White women was 1.2 (10).

Among those women aged 20 years or older who were overweight or obese during the time period from 2013 to 2016, the prevalence of obesity (BMI of 30 or greater) was 56.0 percent among Black women and 37.9 percent among White women. The ratio comparing Black: White women was 1.5 (10).

Obesity (BMI of 30 or greater) in 2018 among women aged 18 years or older was 44.2 percent among Black women and 28.7 percent among White women. The ratio for obesity comparing Black: White women in 2018 was 1.5 (10, 11).

Overweight and obesity among children is of special concern. Obesity and overweight among children may be indicators of a diet high in fat or sugar and of little physical activity. Children who are overweight or obese may develop hypertension or diabetes at young ages. Also, overweight or obesity during childhood increases the risk of cardiovascular disease during adulthood. These underlying conditions may increase the risk of Black female adolescents and young adults for pregnancy complications and enhanced susceptibility to other conditions.

During the period from 2013 to 2018, among children aged 6 to 11 years, the prevalence of obesity among Black females was 24.1 percent. Among White female children aged 6 to 11 years, 10.4 percent were obese during 2013–2018. The ratio comparing obesity among Black female children aged 6–11 years to their White counterparts was 2.3 (10, 11).

Social Determinants of Health and Cardiovascular Disease and Stroke

A number of investigators have explored the associations of exposure to psychosocial stressors with heart disease, and there is a considerable body of research that suggests that social factors, such as exposure to racism and other chronic stressful life conditions, are associated with cardiovascular disease (12). Much of the evidence comes from prospective epidemiologic cohort studies, in which information about social factors and heart disease are assessed at the start of the research. Persons who already have heart disease are excluded. At the end of the research period (or at some point or points in time after enrollment in the research), participants are assessed for onset of cardiovascular disease or death from cardiovascular disease during the study period.

One such investigation is the Black Women's Health Study or BWHS (13). This longitudinal investigation of the health of Black women was initiated in 1995. It was initially funded by the National Cancer Institute (NCI) of the National Institutes of Health (NIH), to enhance the understanding of the etiology of cancer among Black women in the United States (13). Study participants were volunteers recruited from across the United States, using advertisements in magazines (e.g., Essence) and other mechanisms. Ultimately, 59,000 women were enrolled in the research (13). A recent report from the BWHS suggested that perceived interpersonal racism is associated with increased risk for the development of coronary heart disease among Black women in the United States (14).

Several investigations have demonstrated an association between exposure to various chronic social stressors (including interpersonal or structural racism) with elevated blood pressure (15, 16), which increases risk of cardiovascular disease. Results from the Jackson Heart Study demonstrated an association between perceived racial discrimination with increased risk of hypertension among Blacks in the United States (17). Hypertension elevates risk of both cardiovascular disease and stroke.

In addition, there is evidence that living in communities with high levels of social disorganization (such as incarceration, crime, and divorce), especially in combination with poverty, is associated with elevated levels of hypertension among Black adults (18, 19).

Prior research by James and colleagues has demonstrated an association between John Henryism Active Coping (JHAC) style with an increased risk of hypertension among Black adults (20, 21). John Henryism Active Coping is a way of attempting to overcome adversity in the social, economic, and work environment (20, 21). Structural and cultural racism presents barriers to economic and employment success among Blacks in the United States (20, 21). Adults with higher levels of John Henryism struggle to overcome obstacles at work and other situations by working harder to succeed despite the racism that makes their lives difficult. However, the struggle to overcome the structural and cultural racism that is embedded in American society exerts a toll on the health of Blacks. Blacks with higher levels of John Henryism Active Coping have an increased risk of hypertension, and the complications that arise from hypertension, such as cardiovascular disease and stroke (20, 21).

The Black Women's Health Study has also reported that perceived racism (an important type of social stressor) is associated with increased risk of the development of diabetes (22) and with obesity (23). Both diabetes and obesity increase the risk of cardiovascular disease.

Numerous studies have reported that exposure to higher levels of social stressors is associated with depression (24–26). A large body of research has demonstrated associations between depression with cardiovascular disease (27–31) and with stroke (32).

The evidence is clear that cardiovascular disease disproportionately impacts Black compared to White women. Even young Black women have increased risk of cardiovascular disease compared to their White counterparts. Premature death due to cardiovascular disease among Black women during the "prime of life" (ages 15 to 44 years) has tragic outcomes for children and families. Black women are lost during the years when they are mothers raising children, daughters caring for aging parents, and wage earners for their families. Black women in the prime of life also are supportive friends, neighbors, and volunteers in their churches and communities. Many Black women are employed as workers in jobs that are essential to their communities, such as teachers, nurses and other health care workers, and food service workers. Their death creates a void in their families, neighborhoods, churches, and workplaces.

In order to reduce the premature death of young women due to diseases of the heart and stroke, it is necessary to address Social Determinants of Health and to reduce exposure to difficult ongoing social stressors that negatively impact the lives of young Black women. Needed changes will occur through targeted public health approaches (33–37) and interventions (38, 39). These interventions will need to focus upon reducing interpersonal, structural, and cultural racism (36). Exposure to racism is considered to be the underlying cause of racial inequities in health (36). Exposure to other chronic, ongoing social stressors such as poverty, harmful housing, neighborhood, and work conditions, lack of access to good-quality education and health care need to be addressed (36, 37), since these stressors exert a negative influence upon health.

It has been noted that there is not a lack of knowledge about solutions to racial inequities in health, but there is a lack of political will to make the required changes (38, 39). Since cardiovascular disease and stroke are among the leading causes of death among Black women in the United States, achieving health equity by improving the life conditions of Black women is necessary to save countless lives of Black women, and to benefit their children, families, and communities.

References

1 Kyalwazi AN, Loccoh EC, Brewer LC, et al. Disparities in cardiovascular mortality between Black and White adults in the United States. *Circulation* 2022; 146: 211–228.
2 *Health, United States, 2017, with Special Feature on Mortality*. Hyattsville, MD: National Center for Health Statistics, 2018.
3 Heron M. Deaths: leading causes for 2019. *National Vital Statistics Reports; 70 (9)*. Hyattsville, MD: National Center for Health Statistics, 2021.
4 *Health United States, 2019*. Hyattsville, MD: National Center for Health Statistics, 2020.
5 *Health United States, 2015. With Special Feature on Racial and Ethnic Disparities*. Hyattsville, MD: National Center for Health Statistics, 2016.
6 Xu J, Arias E. Deaths: final data for 2019. *Vital Statistics Rapid Release, No. 23*. Hyattsville, MD: National Center for Health Statistics, August 2022.
7 Murphy SL, Kochanek KD, Xu J, Arias E. Mortality in the United States, 2020. *Data Brief 427*. Hyattsville, MD: National Center for Health Statistics, December 2021.
8 Kochanek KD, Xu J, Arias E. Mortality in the United States, 2019. *Data Brief 395*. Hyattsville, MD: National Center for Health Statistics, 2020.

9 Kalinowski J, Taylor JY, Spruill TM. Why are young Black women at high risk for cardiovascular disease? *Circulation* 2019; 139: 1003–1004.
10 *Office of Minority Health: Policy and Data – Minority Population Profiles: Black/African American*. Washington, DC: US Department of Health and Human Services, 2022.
11 *Health, United States 2018*. Hyattsville, MD: National Center for Health Statistics, 2019.
12 Ogunniyi MO, Mahmoud Z, Meusah YC, et al. Eliminating disparities in cardiovascular disease for Black women: JACC review topic of the week. *J Amer Coll Cardiol* 2022; 80: 1762–1771.
13 Palmer JR, Rosenberg L. Research on health disparities: strategies and findings from the Black Women's Health Study. *Am J Epidemiol* 2022; KWAC 022: 1–5.
14 Sheehy S, Brock M, Palmer JR. Abstract P 406: association between perceived racism and incident coronary heart disease among Black women. *Circulation* 2023; 147 (Suppl 1).
15 Lehman BJ, Taylor SE, Kiefe CT, Seeman TE. Relationship of early life stress and psychological function to blood pressure in the CARDIA study. *Health Psychol* 2009; 28: 338–346.
16 Moody DLB, Chang Y, Pantesco EJ, et al. Everyday discrimination prospectively predicts blood pressure across ten years in racially/ethnically diverse mid-life women: study of women's health across the nation. *Ann Behav Med* 2019; 53: 608–620.
17 Forde AT, Sims M, Muntner P, et al. Discrimination and hypertension risk among African-Americans in the Jackson Heart Study. *Hypertension* 2020; 76: 715–723.
18 James SA, Kleinbaum DG. Socioecologic stress and hypertension-related mortality rates in North Carolina. *Am J Public Health* 1976; 66: 354–358.
19 Harberg C, Erfurt JC, Chapel C, et al. Socioecological stressor areas and Black-White blood pressure: Detroit. *J Chr Dis* 1973; 26: 595–611.
20 James SA, Strogatz DG, Wing B, Ramsey DL. Socioeconomic status, John Henryism, and hypertension in Black and White adults. *Am J Epidemiol* 1987; 126: 664–673.
21 Singer J, Sussman N, Martin N, Johnson A. Black men have the shortest lives of any Americans. This theory helps explain why. *Pro Publica*, December 22, 2020.
22 Bacon KL, Staver SO, Cozier YC, et al. Perceived racism and incident diabetes in the Black Women's Health Study. *Diabetologia* 2017; 60: 222–225.
23 Cozier YC, Yu J, Coogan PF, et al. Racism, segregation, and risk of obesity in the Black Women's Health Study. *Am J Epidemiol* 2014; 179: 875–883.
24 Orr ST, James SA, Burns BJ, Thompson B. Chronic stressors and maternal depression: implications for prevention. *Am J Public Health* 1989; 79: 1295–1296.
25 Shah AJ, Velendar E, Hong Y, et al. Depression and history of attempted suicide as risk factors for heart disease mortality in young individuals. *Arch Gen Psychiatry* 2011; 68: 1135–1142.
26 Hammen C. Stress and depression. *Ann Rev Clin Psychol* 2005; 1: 293–319.
27 Lichman JH, Bigger JT, Blumenthal JA, et al. Depression and coronary heart disease. *Circulation* 2008; 118: 1768–1775.
28 Gilmour H. Depression and risk of heart disease. *Health Rep* 2008; 19: 7–18.
29 Bradley SM, Rumsfeld JS. Depression and cardiovascular disease. *Trends Cardiovasc Med* 2015; 25: 614–622.
30 Ford DE, Mead LA, Chang PP, et al. Depression is a risk factor for coronary artery disease in men: the Precursor Study. *Arch Internal Med* 1998; 158: 1422–1426.

31 Pan A, Sun Q, Okereke OI, et al. Depression and risk of stroke morbidity and mortality: a meta-analysis and systematic review. *JAMA* 2011; 306: 1241–1249.
32 Larson SL, Owens PL, Ford D, Eaton W. Depressive disorder, dysthymia, and risk of stroke: 13-year follow-up from the Baltimore Epidemiologic Catchment Area study. *Stroke* 2001; 32: 1979–1983.
33 Smilowitz NR, Maduro GA, Lobach IR, et al. Adverse trends in ischemic heart disease mortality among young New Yorkers, particularly young Black women. *PLoS ONE* 2016; 11: e0149015.
34 James SA. Confronting the moral economy of US racial/ethnic health disparities. *Am J Public Health* 2003; 93: 189.
35 Satcher D, Higginbotham EJ. The public health approach to eliminating disparities in health. *Am J Public Health* 2008; 98 (Suppl): S8–S11.
36 Williams DR, Costa MV, Odunlami AO, Muhammed SA. Moving upstream: how interventions that address the Social Determinants of Health can improve health and racial disparities. *J Public Health Manag Pract* 2008; 14 (Suppl): S8–S17.
37 Williams DR, Purdue-Vaughns V. Needed interventions to reduce racial/ethnic disparities in health. *J Health Polit Policy Law* 2016; 41: 627–651.
38 Miller CA. Societal change and public health: a rediscovery. *Am J Public Health* 1976; 66: 54–60.
39 Weintraub K. Americans' life expectancy continues to fall, erasing health gains of the last quarter century. *USA Today*, December 22, 2022.

6 Malignant Neoplasms (Cancer)

Overview

Malignant neoplasm (cancer) is a leading cause of death among Black and White women. Cancer also causes morbidity, economic strain, inability to work, and inability to fully function as a mother, family member, and member of the community. Cancer treatments are expensive, time-consuming, and can have debilitating side effects.

Mortality From Cancer Among Young, Black Women

Black women have higher mortality rates from cancer overall and for many major sites of cancer compared to White women. Table 6.1 shows cancer mortality rates (age-adjusted per 100,000 population) for Black and White women from 1960 until 2019. As shown in this table, for Black women, cancer mortality (all sites) increased from 1970 until 1990 and then decreased for the period from 2000 until 2019. For White women, cancer mortality also increased from 1970 until 1990 and then decreased for the period 1990 until 2019 (1). The ratios comparing mortality from cancer for Black: White women increased somewhat from 1970 until 1990 and then decreased from 1990 until 2019 (1–10).

Table 6.2 shows mortality from cancer (age-adjusted per 100,000 popu lation) for Black and White women for leading sites of cancer for the years 2014–2020. For many sites of cancer, the mortality among Black women is double that of White women. For example, the age-adjusted mortality per 100,000 population among Black women for Myeloma, cancer of the stomach, and cancer of the uterine corpus is about double that of White women (1). For cancer of the uterine cervix and breast, the age-adjusted mortality per 100,000 population is higher for Black than White women (1).

Cancer Incidence Among Young, Black Women

The racial disparities between Black and White women in cancer incidence are not as great as the disparities in mortality. Table 6.3 shows the cancer incidence (newly diagnosed cases per 100,000 population) for selected sites

DOI:10.4324/9781032663807-6

Table 6.1 Age-Adjusted Mortality per 100,000 Population From Cancer, for Black and White Women, 1950–2019

Year	*Race*		
	White	*Black*	*Ratio Black: White*
1950	182	174.1	0.96
1960	167.7	174.3	1.04
1970	162.5	173.4	1.04
1980	165.2	189.5	1.15
1990	174	205.9	1.18
2000	166.9	193.8	1.16
2013	140.2	158.5	1.13
2014	138.8	156.8	1.13
2019	137.8	150.5	1.1

Source: (References: 1–10)

Table 6.2 Age-Adjusted Mortality per 100,000 Population for Selected Sites of Cancer, Black and White Females, 2016–2020

Site	*Race*		
	Black	*White*	*Ratio Black: White Women*
Breast	27.6	19.7	1.4
Uterine Cervix	3.3	2	1.65
Colon/Rectum	14.3	11.1	1.29
Liver	4.8	3.6	1.35
Myeloma	5	2.2	2.27
Pancreas	12.3	9.6	1.28
Stomach	3.5	1.5	2.31
Uterine Corpus	9.1	4.6	1.98

Source: (References: 2–3, 5–13)

of cancer for Black and White women. For most sites of cancer (with the exceptions of Myeloma and stomach cancer), the ratios for cancer incidence comparing Black: White women are close to 1.0.

Survival From Cancer Among Young, Black Women

In addition to mortality, five-year survival from cancer is an important measure of outcome of cancer. As shown in Table 6.4, overall, for selected sites of cancer, Black women have poorer five-year survival than White women.

Table 6.3 Incidence (New Cases) of Cancer per 100,000 Population for Selected Sites, for Black and White Women, 2014–2018

Site	*Race*		
	Black	*White*	*Ratio Black: White Women*
Uterine Cervix	8.8	7.2	1.22
Colon/Rectum	37.1	31.3	1.18
Liver	5.5	3.9	1.22
Myeloma	12.3	4.8	2.6
Pancreas	15	11.2	1.34
Stomach	7.4	3.5	2.14
Esophagus	2.1	1.8	1.16

Source: (References: 2–5, 10)

Table 6.4 Trends in Five-Year Survival for Selected Sites of Cancer Among Females, by Race, 2011–2017

Site	*Five-Year Survival*	
	Black (%)	*White (%)*
Breast	82	92
Ovary	41	48
Uterine Cervix	56	67
Uterine Corpus	63	84

Source: (Reference: 2)

Table 6.5 shows the lifetime probability of dying from selected cancers for Black and White women. These data are from the American Cancer Society, for the period 2016–2018 (2). It can be seen in this table that Black women have a greater lifetime probability of dying from these cancers than White women.

Stage at Diagnosis of Cancer Among Young, Black Women

The major reason cited for the increased death rate from cancer, and diminished five-year survival, among Black compared to White women, despite the decreased incidence of many cancers, is that Black women tend to be diagnosed with cancer when it is at a more advanced stage than White women. Cancers diagnosed at more advanced stages, when it has metastasized (spread) to other locations in the body, are much harder to cure. This creates a much higher mortality rate and decreased five-year survival.

Table 6.6 shows the stages at diagnosis for several sites of cancer for Black and White women. "Localized" refers to cancers that are restricted to the tumor but have not spread beyond the tumor. "Regionalized" refers to cancers that have spread (metastasized) to surrounding organs, tissues, and lymph nodes beyond the tumor. "Distant" refers to cancers that have spread to organs, tissues, and lymph nodes in other parts of the body, distant from the tumor.

Table 6.6 demonstrates that for several major causes of cancer mortality, Black women are more likely to have their cancers diagnosed at more advanced stages than White women. Cancers diagnosed at later stages, with more spread of the disease beyond the original tumor, are more difficult to successfully treat and to achieve long-term survival.

Table 6.5 Lifetime Probability of Dying From Selected Cancer for Black and White Women, 2016–2018

Cancer Site	*Lifetime Probability of Death*	
	Black Females	*White Females*
Colon and Rectum	1 in 55	1 in 63
Liver	1 in 171	1 in 209
Myeloma	1 in 156	1 in 301
Stomach	1 in 225	1 in 487
Uterine Cervix	1 in 315	1 in 516
Uterine Corpus	1 in 97	1 in 167

Source: (Reference: 2)

Table 6.6 Stage at Diagnosis for Selected Cancers Among Females, by Race, United States, 2014–2018

Cancer and Stage	*Race*	
	Black (%)	*White (%)*
Breast Cancer		
Localized	54	64
Regional	34	27
Distant	9	5
Unstaged	3	3
Cancer of the Uterine Cervix		
Localized	36	44
Regional	25	20
Distant	16	7
Unstaged	7	5
Cancer of the Uterine Corpus		
Localized	53	68
Regional	25	20
Distant	16	7
Unstaged	7	5

Source: (Reference: 2)

As shown in Table 6.7, the five-year survival for various cancers among women is associated with stage at diagnosis. In addition, at each stage of cancer, Black women have poorer five-year survival than White women.

Cancer Screening and Prevention Among Young, Black Women

One reason that Black women are often diagnosed at later stages is that they do not have adequate access to primary and preventive health care (14). As an example, some areas in the United States have been termed "maternity care deserts," due to the lack of providers of reproductive health care (15). The lack of access to primary and preventive health care denies Black women the opportunity to have screening and other tests for various cancers. For example, most deaths from cervical cancer can be prevented if women have cervical cancer screening using Pap smears. Unfortunately, if a Pap smear has a result of possible cancer, then a more expensive follow-up test and treatment (colposcopy) are often required. The lack of screening and appropriate follow-up may partially account for the excess risk of mortality from cervical cancer among Black compared to White women.

In addition, dietary factors, obesity, and overweight are associated with risk of cancer incidence and mortality. Certain vitamins and other nutrients in foods help to prevent cancer, and certain preservatives and food composition (e.g., high-fat content) increase risk of cancer. Yet, some areas and neighborhoods in which Black women live do not have grocery stores with

Table 6.7 Five-Year Survival for Selected Cancers Among Females, by Stage and Race, 2008–2014

Cancer Site and Stage	*Five-Year Survival*	
	Black Women (%)	*White Women (%)*
Breast		
Localized	95	99
Regional	77	86
Distant	20	28
All Stages	81	91
Uterine Cervix		
Local	87	92
Regional	49	57
Distant	11	19
All Stages	56	68
Uterine Corpus		
Local	85	96
Regional	48	71
Distant	9	17
All Stages	62	83

Source: (Reference: 2)

fresh fruits and vegetables and overall healthier foods (16). Moreover, Black women are more likely to be obese or overweight than White women (1).

Summary

In conclusion, data for the United States, for Black and White women, clearly demonstrate higher mortality from cancer for Black compared to White women. Even though Black and White women have about the same risk for the onset of cancer at most sites (incidence), the risk of death from cancer among Black women is higher than that among White women. In addition, for most types of cancer, Black women are less likely than their White counterparts to survive for five years after diagnosis. This is partially attributable to the later stage at diagnosis among Black compared to White women. Once cancer has spread to a site away from the initial tumor, into other organs, tissues, and lymph glands, it is much more difficult to treat and to achieve cure.

Several social factors likely play a role in the increased mortality from cancer among Black compared to White women. First, as noted previously, the exposure of Black women to chronic stressors in the social environment has been shown to be associated with an increased risk of depression (17, 18). Depression has been shown in prior research to be associated with increased risk of cancer (19–22).

Moreover, lack of access to convenient preventive health care services among Black women (due to poverty, lack of public transportation, jobs without time off for medical appointments, lack of health insurance) makes it very difficult for Black women to achieve early diagnosis of cancer. This leads to cancers among Black women to be diagnosed at later stages (regional, distant) than cancers among White women. Cancers diagnosed at later stages have less opportunity for successful treatment (i.e., cure or lengthier survival).

It has also been suggested that Black women may have more aggressive types of breast cancer (23). Specifically, Black women may be more likely to have estrogen and progesterone-negative breast cancers, which are more aggressive, more difficult to treat, and have poorer outcomes (23). Recent research has suggested that women who live in an area that was redlined in the past may be more likely to have more aggressive cancers (24, 25). "Redlining" refers to a government policy, instituted in the 1930s, which allowed banks to discriminate in housing loans. It was legal until 1968 for banks to refuse to make mortgage loans for homes in neighborhoods with higher percentages of Black or low-income residents. This policy had the effect of creating residential segregation (25). Residential segregation continued long after redlining ceased.

The Black Womens' Health Study provides important findings about the associations between exposure to social stressors with cancer. The Black Womens' Health Study, as previously described in Chapter 5, was initiated in 1995, and funded by the National Cancer Institute (NCI) of the National Institutes of Health (NIH). Participants were volunteers, who were recruited using advertisements in magazines (e.g., Essence) and other media of interest to Black women. The study participants (N = 59,000) were followed for decades, after excluding those with certain pre-existing conditions, such as cancer (26).

Among other findings, the Black Womens' Health Study reported that higher levels of life stressors and neighborhood disadvantage were associated with increased risk of breast cancer (27).

Exposure to racism and racial discrimination are individual life stressors that exert a harmful impact on the health of Black women (28, 29). In order to bring about improved health and health equity among Black women in the United States, it will be necessary to reduce exposure to racism, racial discrimination, and other stressors in the social environment of Black women (29–32).

Part of improving the social environment of Black women will involve developing the political will to change social and economic policies that harm Black women in the United States (29–34).

Increased investment in preventive and primary health services for Black women, along with improved access to such services, will likely lead to improved treatment outcomes for cancer among Black women. Reduction of exposure to social stressors, improvement in neighborhood conditions (such as segregation, crowding, crime, and pollution), reduction of poverty, and other improvements in the social environment will likely decrease cancer deaths among Black women.

References

1 Office of Minority Health: Policy and Data – Minority Population Profiles: Black/African American. *US Department of Health and Human Services*, Created 1986. HHS.gov
2 American Cancer Society. *Cancer Facts and Figures for African American/Black People-2022–2024*. Atlanta: American Cancer Society, 2022.
3 *Health, United States, 2017, with Special Feature on Mortality*. Hyattsville, MD: National Center for Health Statistics, 2018.
4 *Health United States, 2015, with Special Feature on Racial and Ethnic Disparities*. Hyattsville, MD: National Center for Health Statistics, 2016.
5 *Health United States, 2019*. Hyattsville, MD, National Center for Health Statistics, 2020.
6 Xu J, Arias E. Deaths: final data for 2019. *Vital Statistics Rapid Release, No. 23*. Hyattsville, MD: National Center for Health Statistics, August 2022.
7 Kochanek KD, Xu J, Arias E. Mortality in the United States, 2019. *National Center for Health Statistics, Data Brief 395*. Hyattsville, MD: National Center for Health Statistics, 2020.
8 Heron M. Deaths: leading causes for 2019. *National Vital Statistics Reports; 70 (9)*. Hyattsville, MD: National Center for Health Statistics, 2021.
9 Surveillance, Epidemiology and End Results Program (SEER), 1975–2009. *Division of Cancer Control and Population Sciences, National Cancer Institute*, 2012.
10 Surveillance, Epidemiology and End Results Program (SEER), 1975–2018. *Division of Cancer Control and Population Sciences, National Cancer Institute*, 2022.

11 Murphy SL, Kochanek KD, Xu J, Arias E. Mortality in the United States, 2020. *Data Brief* 427. Hyattsville, MD: National Center for Health Statistics, December 2021.

12 *Health, United States, 2020–2021*. Hyattsville, MD: National Center for Health Statistics, 2022.

13 Ahmad FB, Anderson RN. The leading causes of death in the United States for 2020. *JAMA* 2020; 325: 1829–1830.

14 Smedley BD, Stith AY, Nelson AR (eds). *Unequal Treatment: Confronting Racial and Ethnic Disparities in Health Care*. Washington, DC: Institute of Medicine, National Academies Press, 2003.

15 *Nowhere to Go: Maternity Care Deserts Across the United States*. Arlington, VA: March of Dimes, 2022.

16 Bower KM, Thorpe RJ, Rohde C, Gaskin DJ. The intersection of neighborhood racial segregation, poverty, and urbanicity and its impact on food store availability in the United States. *Prev Med* 2014; 58: 33–39.

17 Hammen C. Stress and depression. *Ann Rev Clin Psychol* 2005; 1: 293–319.

18 Orr ST, James SA, Burns BJ, Thompson B. Chronic stressors and maternal depression: implications for prevention. *Am J Public Health* 1989; 79: 1295–1296.

19 Shekelle RB, Raynor WJ, Ostfeld AM, et al. Psychological depression and 17-year risk of death from cancer. *Psychosom Med* 1981; 43: 117–125.

20 Gross AL, Gallo JJ, Eaton WW. Depression and cancer risk: 24 years of follow-up of the Baltimore Epidemiologic Catchment Area sample. *Cancer Causes Control* 2010; 21: 191–199.

21 Linkins RW, Comstock GW. Depressed mood and development of cancer. *Am J Epidemiol* 1990; 132: 962–972.

22 Gallo JJ, Armenian HK, Ford DE, et al. Major depression and cancer: the 13-year follow-up of the Baltimore Epidemiologic Catchment Area sample. *Cancer Causes Control* 2000; 11: 751–758.

23 Wright E, Waterman PD, Testa C, et al. Breast cancer incidence, hormone receptor status, historical redlining, and current neighborhood characteristics in Massachusetts, 2005–2015. *JNCI Cancer Spectr* 2022; 6: pkac016.

24 McCullough LE. Long red line: breast cancer incidence at the intersection of unjust structural policies and their contemporary manifestations. *J Nat Cancer Inst Cancer Spectr* 2022; 6: pkac018.

25 Krieger N, Wright E, Chen JT, et al. Cancer stage at diagnosis, historical redlining and current neighborhood characteristics: breast, cervical, lung, and colorectal cancers, Massachusetts, 2001–2015. *Am J Epidemiol* 2020; 189: 1065–1075.

26 Palmer JR, Cozier YC, Rosenberg L. Research on health disparities: strategies and findings from the Black Womens' Health Study. *Am J Epidemiol* 2022; kwac022: 1–5.

27 Barber LE, Zirpoli GR, Cozier YC, et al. Neighborhood disadvantage and individual level life stressors in relation to breast cancer incidence in U.S. Black women. *Breast Cancer Res* 2021; 23: 108.

28 Bailey ZD, Feldman JM, Bassett MT. How structural racism works-racial policies as a root cause of U.S. racial health inequities. *NEJM* 2021; 384: 768–773.

29 James SA. Confronting the moral economy of US racial/ethnic health disparities. *Am J Public Health* 2003; 93: 189.

30 Satcher D., Higgenbotham EJ. The public health approach to eliminating disparities in health. *Am J Public Health* 2008; 98: 400–403.
31 Williams DR, Purdue-Vaughs V. Needed interventions to reduce racial/ethnic disparities in health. *J Health Polit Policy Law* 2016; 41: 627–651.
32 Williams DR, Costa MV, Odunlami AO, Mohammed SA. Moving upstream: how interventions that address the Social Determinants of Health can improve health and reduce disparities. *J Public Health Manag Pract* 2008; 14 (Suppl): S8–S17.
33 Miller CA. Societal change and public health: a rediscovery. *Am J Public Health* 1976; 66: 54–60.
34 Weintraub K. Americans' life expectancy continues to fall, erasing health gains of the last quarter century. *USA Today*, December 22, 2022.

7 Sexually Transmitted Diseases (STDs) and HIV/AIDS

Overview

Sexually transmitted diseases (STDs), which are sometimes called sexually transmitted infections (STIs), are major causes of morbidity in the United States. The United States has among the highest rates of STDs among the higher-income countries (1). The most common sexually transmitted diseases in the United States are Chlamydia trachomatis, Gonorrhea, and Syphilis. These three infections are the focus of this chapter, along with HIV/AIDS.

Each of these common STDs has increased in recent years, a situation termed "out of control" by the National Coalition of STD Directors (2). There have been calls for new prevention and treatment efforts (3). These efforts are especially needed among high-risk groups, such as Blacks and young women.

Data on cases of STDs are obtained from surveillance, which is based upon reports of testing for these conditions in physicians' offices, emergency rooms, hospitals, reproductive health care providers, "urgent care" centers, and other health care providers. The three STDs which are the focus of this chapter are "reportable" conditions, and have Federally funded surveillance programs to identify cases. As cases are identified through laboratory testing, physicians are mandated to report them to the Centers for Disease Control and Prevention (CDC). Of course, undiagnosed cases are not reported, which can lead to underreporting of these diseases.

In 2019, 30.6 percent of cases of Chlamydia trachomatis, Gonorrhea, and Syphilis were diagnosed among Blacks (4), despite Blacks comprising approximately 12 percent of the population of the United States.

Chlamydia Trachomatis

Chlamydia trachomatis is the most common bacterial STD in the United States. It is five times more common among Black women than among White women, as shown next. It increased 2.8 percent in the United States from 2018 to 2019 (4).

DOI:10.4324/9781032663807-7

Chlamydia cases per 100,000 population, Females, 2019, United States by Race
Black females: 1435.7 per 100,000
White females: 274.7 per 100,000
Ratio Black: White females = 5.23

(Reference: 4)

Overall, most cases of Chlamydia are diagnosed among younger people, ages 15–19 years and 20–24 years, as shown in Table 7.1. Approximately 61 percent of cases occur among those 15–24 years of age, which is the segment of the population targeted for screening.

Untreated Chlamydia can cause serious, permanent damage to a woman's reproductive system. It can cause a woman to have difficulty becoming pregnant and can cause ectopic pregnancy, Pelvic Inflammatory Disease (PID), and scarring of the fallopian tubes.

Gonorrhea

Gonorrhea is a very common and treatable STD. As with Chlamydia, Gonorrhea is most common among those 15–24 years of age. In the United States, rates of Gonorrhea among women increased 43 percent from 2015 to 2019 (4). Since 2009, Gonorrhea increased 111 percent, and it increased 5.7 percent from 2019 to 2020 (5). Most of the increase from 2019 to 2020 was among Blacks.

Black women are close to seven times more likely to be diagnosed with Gonorrhea than White women, as shown here.

Cases of Gonorrhea among Women, per 100,000 population, by Race, United States, 2019
Black Females 448.9 per 100,000 population
White Females 65.5 per 100,000 population

Table 7.1 Cases of Chlamydia Trachomatis Among Women, the United States, by Race and Age, 2019

Age (years)	*Reported Cases per 100,000 Population, 2018*		
	Black Females	*White Females*	*Ratio BF:WF*
10–14	251.8	35.9	7.01
15–19	6976.4	1460.1	4.78
20–24	7358.4	1898.6	3.88
25–29	3134.1	722.4	4.34
30–34	1338.9	326.7	4.1
35–39	543	168.4	3.22
40–44	238.3	82.2	2.9

Source: (Reference: 4)

Ratio Black: White Females: 6.9
(Reference: 4)

Rates of reported cases of Gonorrhea are quite high for women aged 15–19 years and 20–24 years, as shown in Table 7.2.

Syphilis

Syphilis is a common sexually transmitted infection, with a 24 percent increase from 2019 to 2020 among women, and a 16 percent increase among pregnant women from 2019 to 2020 (5). Syphilis in a pregnant woman can cause her infant to be born with congenital syphilis, which can lead to health complications or death of newborns.

In 2021, the rate of syphilis was the highest since 1991, and the total number of cases was at the highest level since 1991 (2). Syphilis increased 30 percent among women from 2018 to 2019, and 178.6 percent among women from 2015 to 2019 (4).

Syphilis consists of two stages of infection. Primary syphilis occurs when there is one sore (or a small number of sores), usually in the genital region or mouth. With secondary syphilis, a more widespread rash over other parts of the body occurs, and there may also be fever, headache, and fatigue.

Primary and Secondary syphilis are most common among younger women, ages 20–24 years. As shown in Table 7.3, at all ages from 15 to 44, Black women have an increased risk of syphilis compared to White women.

As with other STDs, syphilis is most common among younger women, as shown in Table 7.3.

Congenital Syphilis occurs through transmission from a pregnant woman infected with syphilis to her baby during childbirth (perinatal transmission). Congenital Syphilis increased 41.4 percent from 2018 to 2019, and 291.1

Table 7.2 Cases of Gonorrhea per 100,000 population Among Females, by Race and Age, United States, 2019

Age (years)	*Race*		
	Black	*White*	*Ratio B: W*
15–19	1794.3	204.9	8.76
20–24	2156	311.9	6.91
25–29	1125.9	220.2	5.11
30–34	570	160.6	3.55
35–39	271.6	103.6	2.62
40–44	139.6	56.7	2.46

Source: (Reference: 4)

Table 7.3 Primary and Secondary Syphilis Cases Per 100,000 Population Among Women, United States, by Race and Age, 2019

Age (years)	*Race*		
	Black	*White*	*Ratio B: W*
15–19	17	2	8.5
20–24	34	5.8	5.86
25–29	28.8	7.1	4.06
30–34	18.7	7.2	2.6
35–39	15.9	5.8	2.74
40–44	10.2	4.4	2.32

Source: (Reference: 4)

percent from 2015 to 2019 (4). Since 2013, Congenital Syphilis has increased each year. Congenital Syphilis occurs with much greater frequency among Black compared to White infants (4).

Reported Cases of Congenital Syphilis, 2019, United States

Blacks: 86.6 per 100,000 live births
Whites: 13.5 per 100,000 live births
Ratio B: W = 6.4
(Reference: 4)

Congenital Syphilis can be prevented by the receipt of routine, regular prenatal care, and by testing pregnant women for syphilis. Women who test positive for syphilis during pregnancy must be properly treated and must comply with treatment.

Prevention of Sexually Transmitted Diseases

The number and rate of reported cases of Chlamydia trachomatous, Gonorrhea, Primary and Secondary Syphilis, and Congenital Syphilis have all risen in the past decade. There are several reasons for the inability to reduce the transmission of these infections, especially among Black women.

First, several aspects of the social environment of Black women increase transmission of STDs. Exposure to chronic, ongoing life stressors increases the risk of depression among women (6, 7). Prior research has clearly demonstrated that women with depression are more likely than women without depression to engage in behaviors that increase the risk of acquiring STDs (8). These behaviors include engaging in intercourse without the use of condoms by their partners and engaging in intercourse with multiple partners.

Also, women who live in neighborhoods in which the rates of STDs are high have a greater risk of having sexual intercourse with an infected partner than women who live in neighborhoods with lower rates of STDs (9, 10).

Many Black women live in neighborhoods in which the rates of STDs are high, increasing their risk of becoming infected.

In order to better control the spread of STDs among Black women, it is necessary that there is access to convenient, accessible sexual health care in the communities in which they live. Testing and treatment must be available, accessible, acceptable, and affordable. There is a need for additional funding for diagnosis and treatment of STDs (11). Delayed diagnosis and treatment, as occurred during the COVID-19 pandemic, increases spread of STDs. There is also a need for new strategies to increase utilization of screening and treatment. With the increases in rates and numbers of STDs in the United States, especially among young Black women, it is clear that increased investment in public health infrastructure to reduce spread and acquisition of STDs is necessary. At the same time, reduction in exposure to social stressors and depression is needed (12–16). Women can also be evaluated for depression and properly treated. This will reduce the infection of Black women with STDs.

HIV/AIDS

In 1981, a small number of cases (five) of a previously unknown infectious condition were reported among men in California (17). The young, previously healthy, gay men all presented for medical care for severe pneumonia. They were all diagnosed with Pneumocystis Carinii pneumonia. The men also had other unusual infections. It appeared that the immune systems of these men were not working properly. The Centers for Disease Control and Prevention (CDC) was alerted to these infections. Four of the five men died very quickly (17).

At about the same time, dermatologists in New York became alarmed about the occurrence of a cluster of cases of a rare and unusually aggressive cancer, Kaposi's Sarcoma (KS), among gay men. KS is associated with weakened immune systems. The CDC was alerted to this cluster of cases of KS in New York (17).

After the CDC reported in *Morbidity and Mortality Weekly Reports* (*MMWR*) about the infections in California and the cases of Kaposi's Sarcoma in New York, cases of unusual infections were reported to the CDC from around the United States. The illnesses all had the common factor of the immune system not functioning properly. The underlying illness became known as Acquired Immunodeficiency Syndrome or AIDS (17, 18).

The infection that caused AIDS was identified as Human Immunodeficiency Virus (HIV), a viral illness transmitted via sexual contact, transfusions of HIV-infected (donated) blood, and shared needles used for injection drug use. HIV can also be transmitted from a pregnant woman to her baby during childbirth. HIV compromises the immune system. It can develop over time into Acquired Immune Deficiency Syndrome (AIDS), which can cause death due to the acquisition of various infections, such as Pneumocystis Carinii pneumonia or opportunistic infections (18).

A task force was created at the CDC to conduct surveillance activities for this new infection and to create a better understanding of HIV in order to control its transmission. However, little funding was allocated to conduct epidemiologic research about HIV. The lack of funding was partially attributable to the stigma of a disease that initially only occurred among gay men. The first substantial funding for HIV was allocated in 1988 (17).

By the early 1990s, a decade after the first cases were reported, there were more than 750,000 people living with HIV in the United States (17). In 1992, AIDS was the leading cause of death among men aged 25–44 years (17).

While the initial cases of HIV and AIDS were among men who had sex with men (MSM), over time, this virus was transmitted to women through heterosexual sexual intercourse, needle sharing, and transfusions of HIV-infected blood. In 2018, Black women accounted for 58 percent of new HIV diagnoses among women, despite comprising only about 12 percent of the female population of the United States. By 2019, the rate of new cases of HIV among Black women was 10.5 times the rate among White women, as shown next. Clearly, HIV disproportionately affected Black compared to White women (20–22).

Rate of New Cases of HIV among Women, by Race, 2019, United States
Black Women: 18.9 cases per 100,000 population
White Women: 1.8 cases per 100,000 population
Ratio Black: White women = 10.5
(Reference: 4)

Also in 2019, cases of AIDS were 15 times higher among Black compared to White women (20.0 per 100,000 population compared to 0.8 per 100,000 population). In 2019, the death rate for HIV for Black women was 6 per 100,000 population, while for White women, the death rate for HIV was 0.8 per 100,000 population. The ratio of the HIV death rates for 2019 comparing Black: White women was 14.5 (23, 24).

By 2020, HIV had become a leading cause of death for Black women. Among Black women aged 25–34 years, HIV was the tenth-leading cause of death. Among Black women aged 35–44 years, HIV was the ninth-leading cause of death. HIV was not among the leading causes of death for White women in these age groups (25, 26).

Despite the large disparities in cases and mortality between Black and White women, overall, the spread of HIV and AIDS was declining, as shown in Table 7.4.

The methods of transmission of HIV were different for Black compared to White women. In 2018, 92 percent of new cases of HIV among Black women were transmitted via heterosexual contact, and 8 percent were transmitted via injection drug use (sharing needles or use of unsterilized needles). Among White women, 64 percent of new cases of HIV were transmitted via

Table 7.4 Cases of HIV per 100,000 population, Among Women, by Race, United States, 1990–2018

Year	*Race*		
	Black	*White*	*Ratio B: W*
1990	26.7	8.3	3.22
2000	23.3	2.8	8.32
2005	19.2	2.2	8.73
2010	11.6	1.4	8.29
2017	6.6	0.9	7.33
2018	6.1	0.9	6.78

Source: (Reference: 24)

heterosexual contact, and 36 percent were transmitted via use of injection drugs (18, 20, 21, 24).

There are several reasons that transmission of HIV is declining. Antiretroviral drugs, which suppress the HIV virus, are given to pregnant women who are infected with HIV to prevent transmission to the baby during childbirth.

Both pre-exposure prophylaxis (PrEP) and post-exposure prophylaxis (PEP) with antiretrovirals are now successfully used to prevent the spread of HIV. However, the use of these medications necessitates both access to health care for HIV-positive persons and access to the medications.

As with other infections transmitted through sexual intercourse, certain behaviors increase the risk of acquiring HIV. These behaviors include having intercourse unprotected by condoms and having multiple partners. In addition, viral suppression through the use of antiretroviral medications requires access to health care and to the medications. Persons who successfully achieve viral suppression (to undetectable levels of virus) can live healthy lives with HIV without progressing to onset of AIDS and will not transmit the virus to sex partners or through perinatal transmission during childbirth.

The goal in the United States is to eliminate the epidemic of HIV/AIDS. The National HIV/AIDS Strategy for 2022–2025 is to end the HIV epidemic by 2030 (27). Black women have been identified by this strategic plan as a priority population.

Placing this within the Social Determinants of Health framework focuses efforts on reducing exposure to social stressors among Black women, such as racism, poverty, and stressors related to employment, neighborhood, and housing (28). Other social factors which enhance transmission of HIV include living in neighborhoods in which the rate of HIV is high. That increases the chances that a sex partner will be infected with HIV. Black women who are already infected with HIV also need to have access to comprehensive health care to obtain appropriate care, including antiretroviral medications so that they can achieve viral suppression.

Reducing racial disparities in health has been termed a "public health challenge of our time" (29). Racism has been identified as the root cause of racial inequities in health (30). In order to address racism as a root cause of health inequities, there is a need to develop the political will to bring about changes in economic and social policies (30–32). By changing social and economic policies, it will be possible to reduce acquisition of STDs and HIV among Black women.

References

1 National Academies of Sciences, Engineering, and Medicine. *Committee on Prevention and Control of Sexually Transmitted Infections in the United States.* Washington, DC: National Academies Press, 2021.
2 "Out of Control" rise in STD's, including 26% syphilis spike, sparks US alarm. *Guardian*, September 20, 2022. (from Associated Press, September 19, 2022).
3 Glenza J. US Sexually transmitted infections surged to record high in 2020. *Guardian*, April 12, 2022.
4 Centers for disease control and prevention, national center for HIV, viral hepatitis, STD, and TB prevention. Sexually transmitted disease surveillance 2019. *Atlanta*, 2020.
5 Centers for disease control and prevention, national center for HIV, viral hepatitis, STD, and TB prevention. Sexually transmitted disease surveillance 2020. *Atlanta*, 2022.
6 Orr ST, James SA, Burns BJ, Thompson B. Chronic stressors and maternal depression: implications for prevention. *Am J Public Health* 1989; 79: 1295–1296.
7 Hammen C. Stress and depression. *Ann Rev Clin Psychol* 2005; 1: 293–319.
8 Orr ST, Celentano DD, Santelli J, Burwell L. Depressive symptoms and risk factors for HIV acquisition among Black women attending urban community health centers in Baltimore. *J AIDS Prev Educ* 1994; 6: 230–236.
9 Lang DL, Salazar LF, Crosby RA, et al. Neighborhood environment, sexual risk behaviors and acquisition of sexually transmitted infections among adolescents diagnosed with psychological disorders. *Am J Community Psychol* 2018; 46: 303–311.
10 Laomann EO, Youm Y. Racial/ethnic group differences in the prevalence of sexually transmitted diseases in the United States: a network explanation. *Sexually Trans Dis* 1999; 26: 250–261.
11 *STI's: National Strategic Plan for the United States: 2021–2025.* Washington, DC: United States Department of Health and Human Services, 2021.
12 Sexually Transmitted Diseases Health Equity. Centers for disease control and prevention. *Atlanta*, 2020.
13 Satcher D, Higgenbotham EJ. The public health approach to eliminating disparities in health. *Am J Public Health* 2008; 98: 400–403.
14 Braveman PA, Arkin E, Proctor D, et al. Systemic and structural racism: definitions, examples, health damage, and approaches to dismantling. *Health Aff* 2022; 41: 171–178.
15 Williams DR, Lawrence JA, Davis BA, Vu C. Understanding how discrimination can affect health. *Health Serv Res* 2019; 54: 1374–1388.
16 Thoits P. Gender and race stress and health: major findings and policy implications. *Am J Prev Med* 2004; 27: 49–56.

17 *A Timeline of HIV and AIDS.* HIVHistory.org
18 *HIV Basics.* HIV.gov.
19 *The HIV/AIDS Epidemic in the United States: The Basics.* San Francisco: Kaiser Family Foundation, June 7, 2021.
20 *Women and HIV in the United States.* San Francisco: Kaiser Family Foundation, March 9, 2020.
21 *Black Americans and HIV/AIDS: The Basics.* San Francisco: Kaiser Family Foundation, February 7, 2020.
22 Bradley ELP, Williams AM, Green S, et al. Disparities in incidence of human immunodeficiency virus among Black and White women – United States, 2010–2016. *Morb Mortal Wkly Rep* 2011; 68 (18): 416–418.
23 Office of Minority Health. *Data and Profile: Population Profiles, Black/African American Health.* US Department of Health and Human Services, 2022.
24 *Health, United States, 2019.* Hyattsville, MD: National Center for Health Statistics, 2020.
25 Murphy SL, Kochanek KD, Xu J, Arias E. Mortality in the United States, 2020. *Data Brief* 427. Hyattsville, MD: National Center for Health Statistics, December 2021.
26 *Health, United States, 2020–2021.* Hyattsville, MD: National Center for Health Statistics, 2022.
27 *National HIV/AIDS Strategy for 2022–2025.* Washington, DC: White House Office on National AIDS Policy, 2022.
28 Williams DR, Costa MV, Odunlami AO, Muhammed SA. Moving upstream: how interventions that address the Social Determinants of Health can improve health and racial disparities. *J Public Health Manag Pract* 2008; 14 (Suppl): S8–S17.
29 Williams DR, Purdie-Vaughns V. Needed interventions to reduce racial/ethnic disparities in health. *J Health Polit Policy Law* 2016; 41: 627–651.
30 James SA. Confronting the moral economy of US racial/ethnic health disparities. *Am J Public Health* 2002; 93: 189.
31 Miller CA. Societal change and public health: a rediscovery. *Am J Public Health* 1976; 66: 54–60.
32 Weintraub K. Americans' life expectancy continues to fall, erasing health gins of the last quarter century. *USA Today*: December 22, 2022.

8 Depression

Overview – Depression Among Women

Depression is a leading cause of disability in the United States and worldwide (1–3). Depression is more common among women than men in the United States. Approximately one in five women in the United States will suffer from depression during her lifetime (4).

The symptoms of depression include sadness, changes in sleep or appetite patterns, fatigue, hopelessness, and lack of pleasure in activities that are usually enjoyable (anhedonia).

A recent nationwide survey of mental health conducted by the Kaiser Family Foundation and CNN found that fully 90 percent of Americans believe that the United States has a mental health crisis (5–7). The mental health crisis associated with the COVID-19 pandemic has been termed the "shadow epidemic" (8). Others have noted that there is an "acute crisis" in mental health among young Blacks in the United States, due to persistent racism and widening disparities in health that were brought to the forefront by the disproportionate deaths and severe illness among Blacks from COVID-19 (9). For example, in 2019, among female students in grades 9–12, Black females were 60 percent more likely to attempt suicide compared to White females in the same grades (10). Pediatricians have termed maternal depression a "Public Health Crisis," due to the negative impact of maternal depression on the health and development of children (11).

Depression Among Women During Pregnancy

The usual age of onset for depression among women is during the childbearing years. The childbearing years (ages 15–44) are the years in which women are pregnant, give birth, and raise children. Depression can have a negative impact upon pregnancy outcome (12–15). Depressed women have greater risk than their counterparts without depression of having a preterm birth outcome or other poor pregnancy outcome (12–15).

DOI:10.4324/9781032663807-8

Depression Among Young Black Women

At one time, the focus on depression among women was largely on White women. However, research in the past several decades has shown that young Black women experience a greater risk of depression than their White counterparts.

Information about risk of depression has been derived from several sources in recent decades in the United States. At one time, the only data available about depression were obtained from inpatient admissions to psychiatric hospitals, and from inferences based on suicides. In the 1960s, the National Institute of Mental Health (NIMH) of the National Institutes of Health (NIH) conducted a study of mental health in the United States. This research, termed the Epidemiologic Catchment Area Study (ECA) provided the first information about depression in community dwelling adults in the United States. Depression was assessed using the Diagnostic Interview Survey or DIS. The DIS was developed by the National Institute of Mental Health. (16). The DIS is a valid and reliable measure of depression, and has been utilized by numerous researchers. The DIS categorizes mental health conditions using diagnostic criteria (16).

The Epidemiologic Catchment Area (ECA) study was conducted in five communities in the United States: New Haven, Connecticut; Baltimore, Maryland; St. Louis, Missouri; Durham, North Carolina; and Los Angeles, California. Data collection occurred from 1980 to 1985.

The ECA study included over 20,000 adults. Among women aged 18–24 years, the six-month prevalence of major depression was higher among Black than White women in all five sites (16).

The next generation of data about depression was obtained from the National Co-morbidity Survey, which was designed to assess not only the prevalence of depression among adults in the United States but also the co-morbidity of multiple mental illnesses, and the co-morbidity of mental illness with substance use. Mental illness and substance use were assessed using the Composite International Diagnostic Interview (or CIDI) (17). Data were collected from 1990 to 1992, from over 8,000 respondents aged 15–54 years. In the age group 35–44 years, Black females had the greatest 30-day prevalence of depression (9.7 percent) of all groups. Among White females aged 35–44 years, the 30-day prevalence of depression was 5.7 percent (ratio Black: White females = 1.7). Among women 25–34 years of age, the 30-day prevalence of depression was 5.6 percent among Blacks and 3.5 percent among Whites (ratio Black: White females = 1.6) (17).

Another large study of depression, the National Survey of American Life, included over 6,000 adults. Data about mental health, exposure to social stressors, physical health, and other factors were collected between 2001 and 2003. Depression was assessed among respondents using the Composite International

Diagnostic Interview (CIDI). Blacks were more likely than Whites to rate their Major Depressive Disorder (MDD) as severe or very severe, and Blacks also labeled their depression as more disabling than Whites (18). In addition, Blacks reported their MDD to have more chronicity than Whites (18).

In another nationwide survey, the Americans' Changing Lives Study (conducted in 1986), over 1,300 adults aged 25–64 years were interviewed about depression using the Center for Epidemiologic Studies Depression Scale (CES-D). Black women were found to have over twice the risk of elevated scores on the CES-D than White women (19). The CES-D was developed by NIMH to assess depression among community-dwelling adults (20). The CES-D contains 20 items, and respondents are asked to indicate the number of days they have experienced each symptom in the past seven days. Symptoms include feelings of sadness, lack of pleasure (anhedonia), changes in appetite, changes in sleep, and crying (20). Scores range from 0 to 60, with a cut-point of 16 or greater used to indicate "significant" symptoms of depression (20). The CES-D has been demonstrated to be reliable and valid and has been utilized in numerous epidemiologic investigations (21–23).

In the large ADD Health Study (National Longitudinal Study of Adolescent to Adult Health), over 20,000 adolescents in grades 7–12 in the 1994–1995 school year were followed into adulthood over five waves of follow-up (24). Depression was assessed using the CES-D.

As was reported from findings of other large nationwide epidemiologic investigations, Black females in the ADD Health Study were found to have a greater risk of depression than White females. Depressive symptoms were highest among women in their late thirties. Black women had a higher level of depressive symptoms compared to White women, and the symptoms of depression lasted for a longer time (i.e., greater chronicity) among Black than White women (24).

In another report, from the National Health and Nutrition Examination Study (NHANES) of the Centers for Disease Control and Prevention, data from 2005 to 2016 demonstrated that the prevalence of depression was higher among Black than White women (25) The NHANES identified depression using the Patient Health Questionnaire or PDQ-9 (26). The NHANES sample included over 31,000 adults aged 20 years or older.

In summary, a number of investigations, which included large samples of Black and White women, found that among young women, Black women had a greater prevalence of depression than White women. This has significant implications for pregnancy outcomes and the health of young Black women.

Depression Among Pregnant and Postpartum Women

Depression among pregnant and postpartum women is of special concern. Prenatal depression has been shown to be associated with increased risk of preterm birth and other poor pregnancy outcomes (12–15). Postpartum depression can have harmful effects upon the health of mothers and their infants. It was reported from the Pregnancy Risk Assessment Monitoring System (PRAMS), a study of prenatal and postpartum health among mothers, which is conducted after they have given birth, that 18.2 percent of Black mothers reported postpartum depression in 2018, compared to 11.4 percent of White mothers (ratio Black: White women = 1.6). Two items to assess depression were developed as part of the PRAMS core questionnaire (27).

Other research has involved samples of women enrolled in clinical settings, usually primary care, prenatal care, or reproductive health care. In one such investigation, involving 1,163 pregnant Black and White women in Eastern North Carolina, Black pregnant women were found to have a 50 percent greater risk of elevated depressive symptoms than White pregnant women after adjustment for age, marital status, and education (28). The mean score on the CES-D in the sample was significantly higher among Black than White pregnant women (28).

In "Suffering in Silence: Mood Disorders Among Pregnant and Postpartum Women of Color," it was reported that overall, Black women during pregnancy and the postpartum period had about twice the risk of depression as White women (29). The title "Suffering in Silence" is partially based upon the stigma associated with mental health problems in the United States. This is particularly true for Black women. There is a stereotype of the "strong Black woman," a caretaker who plays a central and crucial role in her family and community. The "strong Black woman" is not viewed as suffering from chronic and severe fatigue, sadness, and other symptoms associated with depression. Rather, she is central to the social and economic well-being of her family.

Depression and Adult Health

Depression has also been shown in numerous studies of adult health to increase the risk of mortality and morbidity from various conditions, including cancer (30, 31), cardiovascular disease (32–36), stroke (37), and hypertension (38). Pregnant women with higher levels of depressive symptoms are more likely to report being in poorer health and functional status than women with lower levels of depressive symptoms (39), and to smoke during pregnancy (40, 41).

Summary

Depression is a serious, common, debilitating, and chronic mental health condition among young Black women. Reasons for the increased risk of depression among Black compared to White women include exposure to racial discrimination and exposure to chronic social stressors over the life course (42–45).

In each of the studies reviewed, which included large, nationwide samples of women and smaller samples obtained in prenatal and pediatric providers of health care, young Black women had a greater risk of depression than their White counterparts. Some samples included pregnant women. Depression among pregnant women is associated with increased risk of poor pregnancy outcomes, poorer self-reported health status, and increased risk of smoking during pregnancy compared to women without depression.

These findings make it clear that the United States, to improve the health of the nation, and especially Black women and families, must develop the public health infrastructure to identify and treat depression (46, 47). Women receiving prenatal, postpartum, or reproductive health care should be screened for depression (48). Similarly, mothers bringing children for pediatric care can be screened for depression (11). Women found to have depression should be referred for treatment.

While the American College of Obstetrics and Gynecology (ACOG) (48) and other organizations (e.g., the American Academy of Pediatrics (11)) recommend screening women for depression, or asking them about symptoms of depression, this is often not done (49). The US Preventive Services Task Force recommends screening all adults for depression and referring depressed adults for appropriate treatment (50, 51). Recognition of depression and referral for treatment would likely benefit the health of infants, children, and mothers.

Also, in order to reduce the risk of depression of Black women, it is necessary to identify and reduce those factors that increase risk of depression. These factors include exposure to stressors in the social environment (such as racism, poverty, economic, housing, and employment instability, and neighborhood deficiencies). Improving the lives of depressed women will improve the health and well-being of depressed women, as well as their children and families.

References

1 Friedrich MJ. Depression is the leading cause of disability around the world. *JAMA* 2017; 317: 1517.

2 Murray CA, Lopez AD. Alternative projections of mortality and disability by cause 1990–2020: Global Burden of Diseases Study. *Lancet* 1997; 349: 1498–1504.

3 The US Burden of Disease Collaborators. The state of US health, 1990–2016. Burden of diseases, injuries and risk factors among US states. *JAMA* 2018; 319: 1444–1472.

4 Weissman MM, Olfson M. Depression in women: implications for health care research. *Science* 1995; 269: 799–801.

5 Palosky C. *New Kaiser Family Foundation/ CNN Survey on Mental Health Finds Young Adults in Crisis: More Than a Third Say Their Mental Health Keeps them from Doing Normal Activities*. San Francisco: Kaiser Family Foundation, October 6, 2022.

6 Lopes L, Kirzinger A, Sparks G, et al. *Kaiser Family Foundation/CNN Mental Health in America Survey*. San Francisco: Kaiser Family Foundation, October 5, 2022.

7 McPhillips D. 90 % of U.S. adults say U.S. is experiencing a mental health crisis, *CNN/KFF Poll Finds*. San Francisco: Kaiser Family Foundation, October 5, 2022.

8 Owens C. America's shadow epidemic. *Axios*, October 30, 2021.
9 Jones C. Black youths face rising rates of depression, anxiety, suicide. *EdSource*, January 25, 2022.
10 *Office of Minority Health. Policy and Data: Blacks/African Americans*. Washington, DC: United States Department of Health and Human Services, 2022.
11 Goeglein SK, Yatchmink YE. Maternal depression is a public health crisis: the time to act is now. *Pediatrics* 2020; 146: e2020010413.
12 Orr ST, James SA, Blackmore-Prince C. Maternal prenatal depressive symptoms and spontaneous preterm birth among African American women in Baltimore, MD. *Am J Epidemiol* 2002; 156: 792–802.
13 Hoffman S, Hatch MC. Depressive symptomatology during pregnancy: evidence for an association with decreased fetal growth in pregnancies of lower social class women. *Health Psychol* 2000; 19: 535–543.
14 Gavin AR, Chae DH, Mustillo S, Liefe CI. Prepregnancy depressive mood and preterm birth in Black and White women: findings from the CARDIA study. *J Womens Health* 2008; 18: 803–811.
15 Staneeva A, Bogossian F, Pritchard M, Witt-Kowalski A. The effects of maternal depression, anxiety, and perceived stress during pregnancy on preterm birth: a systematic review. *Women Birth* 2015; 28: 179–193.
16 Somervell PD, Leaf PJ, Weissman MM, Blazer DG, Bruce ML. The prevalence of ECA/DIS major depression in Black and White adults in five US communities. *Am J Epidemiol* 1989; 130: 725–735.
17 Blazer DG, Kessler C, McGonagle K, Swartz M. The prevalence and distribution of major depression in a national community sample: the National Comorbidity Survey. *Am J Psychiatr* 1994; 151: 979–986.
18 Williams DR, Gonzalez HM, Neighbors H, et al. National Survey of American Life. *Arch Gen Psychiatr* 2007; 64: 305–315.
19 Gazmararian JA, James SA, Lepkowski JM. Depression in Black and White women: the role of marriage and socioeconomic status. *Ann Epidemiol* 1995; 5: 455–463.
20 Radloff LS. The CES-D scale: a self-report depression scale for research in the general population. *Appl Psychol Meas* 1977; 1: 385–401.
21 Roberts RE. Reliability of the CES-D scale in different ethnic contexts. *Psychiatr Res* 1980; 2: 125–134.
22 Husaini BA, Neff JA, Harrington JB, et al. Depression in rural communities: validating the CES-D scale. *J Comm Psychol* 1980; 8: 20–27.
23 Weissman MM, Sholomskas D, Pottenger M, et al. Assessing depressive symptoms in five psychiatric populations: a validation study. *Am J Epidemiol* 1977; 106: 203–214.
24 Udry R. *Depressive symptoms in the National Longitudinal Study of Adolescent to Adult Health (ADD Health). Carolina Population Center*. Chapel Hill: University of North Carolina, 2022, 1.
25 Iranpour S, Sabour S, Kochi F, Saadati HM. The trend and pattern of depression prevalence in the United States: data from the National Health and Nutrition Examination Survey (NHANES) 2005–2016. *J Affect Dis* 2002; 298: 508–515.
26 Kronke K, Spitzer RL, Williams JB. The PHQ-9: validity of a brief depression severity measure. *J Gen Inter Med* 2001; 16: 606–613.

27 Taylor J, Gamble CM. *Mood Disorders Among Pregnant and Postpartum Women of Color*. Washington, DC: Center for American Progress, November 17, 2017.
28 Orr ST, Blazer DG, James SA. Racial disparities in elevated prenatal depressive symptoms among Black and White women in Eastern North Carolina. *Ann Epidemiol* 2006; 16: 463–468.
29 Taylor J, Gamble CM. *Suffering in Silence: Mood Disorders Among Pregnant and Postpartum Women of Color*. Washington, DC: Center for American Progress, November 17, 2017.
30 Gross AL, Gallo JJ, Eaton WW. Depression and cancer risk: 24 years of follow-up of the Baltimore ECA sample. *Cancer Causes Control* 2021; 2: 191–199.
31 Gallo JJ, Armenian HK, Ford DE, et al. Major depression and cancer: the 13-year follow-up of the Baltimore Epidemiologic Catchment Area study sample. *Cancer Causes Control* 2000; 11: 151–158.
32 Gaffey AE, Cavanaugh CE, Rosman L, et al. Depressive symptoms and incident heart failure in the Jackson Heart Study: differential risk among Black men and women. *J Am Heart Assoc* 2022; 11: e022514.
33 Gilmour H. Depression and risk of heart disease. *Health Rep* 2008; 19: 7–17.
34 Meyer CM, Armenian HK, Eaton WW, Ford DE. Incident hypertension associated with depression in the Baltimore Epidemiologic Catchment Area follow-up study. *J Affect Dis* 2004; 83: 127–133.
35 Ferketich AK, Schwartzbaum JA, Frid DJ, et al. Depression as an antecedent to heart disease among women and men in the NHANES study. *Arch Int Med* 2000; 160: 1261–1268.
36 Anda R, Williamson D, Jones D, et al. Depressed affect, hopelessness, and the risk of ischemic heart disease in a cohort of U.S. adults. *Epidemiol* 1993; 4: 285–294.
37 Dong J-Y, Zhang Y-H, Tong J, et al. Depression and risk of stroke. *Stroke* 2012; 43: 32–37.
38 Davidson K, Jonas BS, Dixon KE, et al. Do depression symptoms predict early hypertension incidence in young adults in the CARDIA study? *Arch Gen Int Med* 2000; 160: 1495–1500.
39 Orr ST, Blazer DG, James SA, Reiter JP. Depressive symptoms and indicators of maternal health status during pregnancy. *J Women's Health* 2007; 16: 535–542.
40 Orr ST, Newton ER, Tarwater PM, Weismiller DG. Factors associated with prenatal smoking among Black women in Eastern North Carolina. *Mat Child Health J* 2005; 9: 245–252.
41 Orr ST, Newton ER, Weismiller DG. Prenatal smoking cessation among Black and White women in Eastern North Carolina. *Am J Health Promot* 2007; 21: 192–195.
42 Orr ST, James SA, Burns BJ, Thompson B. Chronic stressors and maternal depression: implications for prevention. *Am J Public Health* 1989; 79: 1295–1296.
43 Quist AJL, Baird DD, Wise LA, et al. Life course racism and depressive symptoms among young Black women. *J Urban Health* 2022; 99: 55–66.
44 Williams DR. Stress and the mental health of populations of color: advancing our understanding of race-related stressors. *J Health Soc Behav* 2018; 59: 466–485.
45 Hammen C. Stress and depression. *Ann Rev Clin Psychol* 2005; 1: 293–319.
46 Bailey RK. The social determinants of mental health. *Am J Psychiatr* 2015; ajp.2015.15040450.

47 Bailey RK, Mokonogho J, Kumar A. Racial and ethnic differences in depression: current perspectives. *Neuropsychiatr Dis Treat* 2019; 15: 603–609.
48 Committee on Obstetric Practice. Screening for perinatal depression. American College of Obstetrics and Gynecology Opinion Number 757. *Obstet Gynecol* 2018; 132: e208–e212.
49 Bauman BL, Ko JY, Cox S, et al. Vital Signs: postpartum depressive symptoms and provider discussions about perinatal depression – United States, 2018. *Morb Mortal Wkly Rep* 2020; 69 (19): 575–581.
50 United States Preventive Services Task Force. Screening for depression: recommendations and rationale. *Ann Inter Med* 2002; 136: 760–764.
51 United States Preventive Services Task Force. Screening for depression in adults: recommendation statement. *Am Fam Phys* 2016; 94: published online August 15, 2016.
52 Brown TN, Williams DR, Jackson JS, et al. "Being black and feeling blue": the mental health consequences of racial discrimination. *Race Soc* 2000; 2: 117–131.

9 Homicide

Homicide as a Public Health Problem Among Young, Black Women

Every day in the United States in 2020, five Black women were killed. There was a 33 percent increase in the rate of homicide among Black women and girls from 2019 to 2020 (1–3). Among White women, from 2019 to 2020, the increase in homicide was 15 percent (1–3). Homicides among Black women are at the highest level since 1994 (1–3). Each of these deaths creates a void in Black families, neighborhoods, communities, and churches.

Homicide is often considered a public health problem that impacts primarily young Black males, but this is not true. Homicide in the Black community is a significant problem for young women as well. In addition, Black women have a substantially greater risk of homicide compared to White women. In 2020, Black women had four times the risk of being homicide victims as White women, as shown next (4).

Age-Adjusted Rates of Homicide per 100,000 population among Women, by Race, United States, 2020
Black women: 8.0
White women: 2.0
Ratio Black: White women = 4
(Reference: 4)

The increased risk of homicide for Black compared to White women has been a public health problem for over half a century, as shown in Table 9.1.

Overall, homicide occurs with greater frequency among both Black and White women aged 25–44, compared to those aged 15–24, as shown in Table 9.2. However, for each age group, Black women are more likely to be victims of homicide than White women.

In 2019, as shown in Table 9.3, age-adjusted homicide mortality was much higher among Black than White women. The highest mortality rates among Black women were among those women aged 20–24 years. In the two youngest groups of women (ages 15–19 and 20–24 years), Black women had approximately seven times the risk of homicide than White women.

DOI:10.4324/9781032663807-9

Table 9.1 Age-Adjusted Homicide Rates per 100,000 Population Among Women by Race, United States 1950–2020

Year	*Race*		
	White	*Black*	*Ratio B: W*
1950	1.4	11.1	7.93
1960	1.5	11.4	7.6
1970	2.3	14.7	6.39
1980	3.2	13.2	4.13
1990	2.7	12.5	4.63
2000	2.1	7.1	3.38
2010	1.8	5	2.78
2014	1.7	4.7	2.76
2016	1.9	5.7	3
2020	2	8	4

Source: (References: 1–3, 6–11)

Table 9.2 Homicide Rates per 100,000 Population by Age and Race Among Females, United States, 1950–2014

Year	*Race and Age*			
	White		*Black*	
	15–24 years	*25–44 years*	*15–24 years*	*25–44 years*
1950	1.3	2	16.5	22.5
1960	1.5	2.1	11.9	22.7
1970	2.7	3.3	17.7	25.3
1980	4.7	4.2	18.4	22.6
1990	4	3.8	18.9	21
2000	2.7	2.9	10.7	11
2010	2	2.4	7.5	7.4
2014	1.7	2.3	7	6.7

Source: (Reference: 6)

Moreover, homicide was the second-leading cause of death for young (ages 15–19 years and 20–24 years) Black women. For White women in these age groups, homicide was the fourth-leading cause of death (5). These data suggest that homicide is a more significant health problem among Black than White women.

Overall, among Black women over 18 years of age, close to 40 percent of homicides during 2003–2014 occurred among women aged 18–29 years, as shown in Table 9.4. Among White women, 21.4 percent of homicides occurred among women aged 18–29 years. Over 60 percent of homicides among Black women occurred among those aged 18–39, while among White women, approximately 40 percent of homicides occurred among women aged 18–39 years (12). (These data are from 18 states.)

The death of young women, under age 40 and during the "prime of life," creates a void in Black families, when these women are mothers caring for children, daughters caring for parents, sisters, wives, neighbors, members of churches and community organizations, and economic providers.

Thus, as shown in Table 9.4, among Black women, homicide affects younger women more than older women.

Homicide Among Young, Black Women and Interpersonal Violence

Additionally, 18.6 percent of female Black homicide victims during the period 2003–2014 were pregnant or six weeks or less postpartum. Among White female homicide victims, 12.92 percent were pregnant or six weeks or less postpartum. Over one-half of both White and Black female homicide

Table 9.3 Age-Adjusted Mortality per 100,000 Population From Homicide Among Women, by Age and Race, and Rank as Leading Cause of Death, United States, 2019

Age (years)	*Race*		
	Black	*White*	*Ratio B: W*
15–19	8.9 (2nd-leading cause)	1.2 (4th-leading cause)	7.42
20–24	14.2 (2nd-leading cause)	2.1 (4th-leading cause)	6.76
25–34	10 (4th-leading cause)	2.3 (5th-leading cause)	4.35
35–44	8.4 (5th-leading cause)	2.5 (8th-leading cause)	3.36

Source: (References: 5, 7)

Table 9.4 Age Distribution of Homicides Among Women Aged 18 years or Older, by Race, 2003–2014, United States

Age (years)	*Race*	
	White (%)	*Black (%)*
18–29	21.40	38.70
30–39	19.00	23.60
40–49	21.60	20.00
50–59	15.80	10.00
60 +	22.10	7.70

Source: (Reference: 12)

victims were killed with firearms during the period from 2003 to 2014 (Black women: 57.7%; White women: 53.4%) (12). In 2020, 75 percent of Black female homicide victims were killed with a firearm (13–14).

Among Black women who are victims of homicide, the relationship of the victim to her killer is unknown in 45 percent of homicides. Among White women, the relationship of the homicide victim to her killer is unknown in only 22 percent of cases. This is partially due to silence about female homicide in the Black community (2). Black women are viewed as caretakers and pillars of the community, not as victims of violence. Rising homicide rates among young Black women have been termed an "unspoken epidemic" (3).

Homicide Among Young, Black Women and Social Determinants of Health

One author calls the United States a "death trap due to guns, drugs, cars and disease" (15). These factors can best be addressed by focusing on "upstream" interventions, such as gun control legislation. These factors (guns, drugs, cars, and disease) are major contributors to shortened life expectancy in the United States compared to other high-resource nations. They are determined largely through policies and social factors (15).

Focusing on Social Determinants of Health (SDOH), it is possible to better understand and control homicide among Black women. For example, changes in laws and policies about the sale, safety, and storage of guns would lead to a reduction in homicides related to gun ownership and guns in the home.

In addition, exposure to chronic social stressors related to economic, housing, and neighborhood instability is associated with increased risk of violence (13). Reduction of exposure to chronic social stressors could lead to a reduction in violence, including firearm-related deaths. Gun violence increased more in recent years in those neighborhoods with higher levels of poverty (1–3). Social programs to decrease poverty would very likely lead to diminished gun violence and homicide.

About 40 percent of homicides among Black women are precipitated by arguments or jealousy involving an intimate partner (12). Programs to promote positive social interactions may lead to decreased violence and homicide (14).

Summary

Homicide among young Black women is a significant public health problem, and one that often is unrecognized. Rates of homicide among Black women are at the highest level since 1994. The pandemic of COVID-19 likely contributed to the increase in homicide among Black women, by exacerbating social stressors such as economic instability, and death and illness among family members. In addition, killings of Black Americans by police (such as George Floyd and Breonna Taylor) during the pandemic increased awareness of racial discrimination in the United States, which is a significant, important social stressor (16).

By addressing the Social Determinants of Health, focusing on exposure to chronic, ongoing social, economic, neighborhood, and health-related stressors, it may be possible to reduce homicides among Black women.

In addition, changes in policies and laws involving firearms are necessary upstream factors to reduce firearm-related homicides among Black women (17).

References

1 Beckett L, Clayton A. At least 4 Black women and girls were murdered per day in the United States last year. *Guardian*, October 6, 2021.

2 Beckett L, Clayton A. An "unspoken epidemic": homicide rate increases for Black women rivals that of Black men. *Guardian*, July 29, 2022.

3 Beckett L, Clayton A. The killing of Black women: five findings from our investigation. *Guardian*, June 30, 2022.

4 Murphy SL, Kochanek KD, Xu J, Arias E. Mortality in the United States 2020. *Data Brief 427*. Hyattsville, MD: National Center for Health Statistics, December 2021.

5 Kochanek KD, Xu J, Arias E. Mortality in the United States 2019. *Data Brief 395*. Hyattsville, MD: National Center for Health Statistics, 2020.

6 *Health, United States, 2015, with Special Feature on Racial and Ethnic Disparities*. Hyattsville, MD: National Center for Health Statistics, 2016.

7 *Health, United States, 2019*. Hyattsville, MD: National Center for Health Statistics, 2020.

8 *Health, United States, 2017. With Special Feature on Mortality*. Hyattsville, MD: National Center for Health Statistics, 2018.

9 *Health, United States, 2020–2021*. Hyattsville, MD: National Center for Health Statistics, 2022.

10 Leading Causes of Death- Females – Non-Hispanic Black, United States, 2018. *National Vital Statistics Rep 2021; 70 (4)*. Hyattsville, MD, May 17, 2021.

11 Leading Causes of Death- Females – Non-Hispanic White, United States, 2018. *National Vital Statistics Rep 2021; 70 (4)*. Hyattsville, MD, May 17, 2021.

12 Petrosky E, Blair JM, Betz CJ, et al. Racial and ethnic differences in homicides of adult women and the role of interpersonal violence. *Morb Mortal Wkly Rep* 2017; 66 (28): 741–746.

13 Kegler SR, Dahlberg LL, Vivolo-Kantor AM. A descriptive exploration of the geographic and sociodemographic concentration of firearm homicide in the United States, 2004–2018. *Am J Prev Med* 2021; 153: 106767.

14 Kegler SR, Simon TR, Zwald ML. Vital Signs: changes in firearm homicide rates- United States, 2019–2020. *Morb Mortal Wkly Rep* 2022; 71 (19): 656–663.

15 Thompson D. America is a rich death trap. *Atlantic*, September 7, 2022.

16 Galea S, Abdella SM. COVID-19 pandemic, unemployment, and civil unrest- Underlying deep racial and socioeconomic divides. *JAMA* 2020; 324: 227–228.

17 Williams DR, Costa MV, Odunlami AO, Mohammed SA. Moving upstream: how interventions that address the Social Determinants of health care can improve health and racial disparities. *J Public Health Manag Pract.* 2008; 14 (Suppl): S8–S17.

10 Health Care

Health of Young Black Women

Young Black women have much poorer health status than young White women. As previously described in the chapters of this book, the mortality from a variety of causes, including cardiovascular disease, cerebrovascular disease, homicide, maternal (pregnancy-related) mortality, AIDS, cancer, and, most recently, COVID-19, is much greater among young Black than young White women. Black women have diminished life expectancy at birth compared to White women. In addition, all-cause, age-adjusted mortality is greater among Black than White women (1–11).

Moreover, morbidity from sexually transmitted infections, depression, hypertension, diabetes, overweight and obesity, and severe maternal morbidity of pregnancy is greater among young Black than White women (1–6). Black women are more likely than White women to describe themselves as in "fair or poor" health than White women (12).

These indicators demonstrate the poorer health status of Black compared to White women. Overwhelmingly, Black women bear a disproportionate burden of multiple physical and mental health conditions compared to their White counterparts. These disparities can be interpreted to indicate a greater need for health care among Black compared to White women, even at young ages. Despite improvements in health among young Black women over the past century, racial inequities remain and need to be addressed.

The United States spends more per capita on health care than most other high-resource nations. Despite the high level of spending on health care, the United States has poorer health outcomes than other wealthy nations (13). It has been estimated that only 10–20 percent of health outcomes in the United States can be attributed to health care (14). Social, economic, political, neighborhood, employment, and environmental conditions are largely responsible for health outcomes in the United States. Yet, health care is needed to prevent, diagnose, and treat various conditions.

DOI:10.4324/9781032663807-10

Access and Barriers to Health Care by Black Women

The Institute of Medicine published a book close to 20 years ago entitled *Unequal Treatment*, which was focused upon problems with the receipt of health care by Blacks in the United States (15). Sadly, there remain many difficulties that face Black women seeking health care. White women do not face many of these difficulties. One author noted, commenting about the experiences of Black women with the health care system, "You Learn to Go Last." This author described beliefs of Black women who received health care in Milwaukee, Wisconsin, and who participated in focus groups (16). The women described perceived discrimination within the health care system in three areas: insurance/income, race, and lifetime experiences of discrimination based on race or poverty. The women also reported that they were treated differently than White women by staff and health care providers (16).

The causes of the health inequities between young Black and White women are found, for the most part, outside the health care system. The exposure of Black women to uncontrollable, toxic, chronic, stressful life conditions ages them prematurely and causes premature death compared to White women (17–20).

Black women often face racism when trying to access health care. Even though this book is about young Black women, a story about a male scientist at the CDC illustrates how discrimination can negatively impact the health of Blacks in the United States. The story is from the summer of 2022. The scientist, Dr. William L. Jeffries IV, earned a Ph.D. in Sociology and was trained to investigate infectious disease outbreaks in the elite Epidemic Intelligence Service (EIS) at the CDC. He works in Atlanta, as a senior scientist in the CDC Office of Health Equity, Division of HIV Prevention. In July 2022, Jeffries developed chills, fever, and sores on his body suggestive of the onset of Monkeypox. Cases of Monkeypox had recently been detected in the United States, mainly among gay men. He was very uncomfortable and in pain, so sought care at a local walk-in health clinic. Unfortunately, the clinic did not have the test for Monkeypox available, nor treatment. Still in pain, he sought care at the Emergency Room of the Emory University Hospital. He found no testing or treatment there, either. Frustrated, sick, and in pain, he called a colleague at the CDC, who was leading the CDC response to Monkeypox.

The burden of Monkeypox fell disproportionately on Blacks, especially gay Black men like Dr. Jeffries. Jeffries was becoming angry at the difficulties he was experiencing obtaining care. He realized that if he, a trained public health scientist who worked at the Nation's premier public health agency, had this much difficulty obtaining testing and treatment, what sort of problems were other gay Black men with Monkeypox experiencing?

Jeffries' friend at the CDC was able to secure an appointment for him with an infectious disease specialist at Emory for the same day. He was admitted to the hospital and received treatment for Monkeypox and for pain.

At the time, Georgia had the second-largest number of cases of Monkeypox in the nation. Three-quarters of the cases occurred among Blacks. Many of the cases were already infected with HIV. Many new diseases strike the Black community first, due to factors that increase susceptibility to disease, such as underlying health conditions, poverty, and overcrowded living conditions.

Jeffries had to seek care for Monkeypox at three different sites. Testing and treatment were unavailable at the first two places. There was a delay across the country in making testing, treatment, and vaccines available. It has been suggested that racism was responsible for the slow response to the outbreak of Monkeypox. Early in the outbreak, little funding was available to control spread of the disease. State health departments had to use funds from STD control and other programs to try to stem the spread of Monkeypox. Cases began to decrease, due to availability of vaccine doses, testing, and behavior change. Jeffries was released from the hospital and recovered. He remains angry at the structural racism, which created such difficulties for him to find testing and treatment (21). The same type of factors (racism, barriers to care, lack of access to care) create problems for Black women to find appropriate health care for pregnancy, depression, cancer, and other health conditions.

One of the greatest needs for health care among young Black women is for reproductive health care, including prenatal care. Information from many sources demonstrates that Black women are more likely than their White counterparts to receive late or no prenatal care (22). Health care is also needed for women prior to becoming pregnant, since women with underlying health conditions such as hypertension have an increased risk of having a preterm birth, complications of pregnancy, or other poor pregnancy outcomes (23, 24). Reproductive health care is also needed by women to help prevent unintended pregnancies. Black women are more likely than White women to have unintended pregnancies (25). Women with unintended pregnancies have a greater risk of preterm birth than women with intended pregnancies (26).

It has been shown that there are areas in the United States in which there are no providers of prenatal or obstetric care. These areas are termed "maternity care deserts" (27). Maternity care deserts are often located in rural or low-income areas, in which Black women are more likely to live than White women.

Black women are more likely than White women to lack health insurance, to have jobs that do not have paid sick leave to go to appointments for health and mental health care, and to not have a regular source of health care. It has been suggested that children and others need a "medical home," where health care is coordinated, and patients are treated with dignity and respect (28). In addition, the high cost of many medications forces Black women to take reduced doses of prescription medications that are needed to maintain their health (e.g., cutting pills in half or skipping days) (29, 30). Medication adherence is an important aspect of treatment for many illnesses (29).

Racism impacts the health of Black women in other ways. Negative stereotypes among White physicians result in young Black women being treated with lack of dignity and respect (31). The symptoms reported and described by young Black women are often dismissed. These dismissals can cost Black women their lives, as described in Chapter 3. CDC Epidemiologist Dr. Shalom Irving died in the days after she gave birth because her symptoms and reports of edema and pain in the days after giving birth were not taken seriously by her physicians (32).

Another paper describes the racism of physicians causing them to view a Black, pregnant woman as "incompetent," due to her race (33).

The communication between White physicians and young Black women is often not positive or culturally sensitive. It has been suggested that implicit bias or racism by health care providers influences medication adherence, physician/patient communication, and patient outcome (31).

These inequities in access to and receipt of health care contribute to the diminished health status of young Black women compared to young White women. In order to improve the health of young Black women, it is necessary to take steps to make changes to the delivery of health care to young Black women.

Needed Changes to Improve the Delivery of Health Care to Young, Black Women

Many groups, including the American Academy of Pediatrics, the American College of Obstetrics and Gynecology, and the United States Preventive Services Task Force, concur that it is important to address the need for mental health care among Black women, especially those who are pregnant, postpartum, or mothers of young children (34–37). Women should be screened for mental health or substance use problems and referred for treatment when needed. The White House Blueprint for Addressing the Maternal Health Crisis in the United States (from June 2022) includes addressing mental health and substance use problems in their recommendations (38).

There is also a need to reduce barriers to health care among young Black women, such as long waiting times for care, complex bureaucracy to navigate, and lack of positive communication between patients and providers.

It has also been suggested to take a broad public health approach to the provision of health care to young, Black women. This approach emphasizes the links between health with social, economic, and environmental disadvantage (17, 39). Improving the health of young, Black women requires addressing all the social determinants of health, including health care.

Importantly, it is imperative to recognize and eliminate the structural and systemic racism within the health care system that negatively impacts the health of young, Black women. Black women bear a disproportionate burden of many health conditions, and difficulties with barriers and access to health care magnify these inequities. While the underlying causes of many health problems are found outside the health care system, there is a clear role for health care to provide necessary services to improve and protect the health of young, Black women, such as preventive care (e.g., immunizations), screening for early identification of health problems, diagnostic testing (e.g., for Monkeypox, sexually transmitted infections, and COVID-19), and equity in access to proper therapies.

It is time for Americans, using their votes and voices, to eliminate health inequities. This will require improving the delivery of health care to Black women, providing health-enhancing resources, and removing exposure to racism and other social stressors over the life course of Black women.

References

1 *Health United States 2015: With Special Feature on Racial and Ethnic Disparities*. Hyattsville, MD: National Center for Health Statistics, 2016.
2 Mahajan S, Caraballo C, Lu Y, et al. Trends in differences in health status and health care access and affordability by race and ethnicity in the United States, 1999–2018. *JAMA* 2021; 326: 637–648.
3 *Health, United States, 2017, With Special Feature on Mortality*. Hyattsville, MD: National Center for Health Statistics, 2018.
4 *Health, United States, 2019*. Hyattsville, MD: National Center for Health Statistics, 2020.
5 *Health, United States, 2020–2021*. Hyattsville, MD: National Center for Health Statistics, 2022.
6 Office of Minority Health. *Policy and Data Profile: Black/African American Health*. Washington, DC: United States Department of Health and Human Services, 2023.
7 Arias E, Tejada-Vera B, Ahmad F, Kochanek KD. Provisional life expectancy estimates for 2020. *Vital Statistics Rapid Release, No. 15*. Hyattsville, MD: National Center for Health Statistics, July 2021.
8 Arias E, Tejada-Vera B, Kochanek KD, Ahmad FB. Provisional life expectancy estimates for 2021. *Vital Statistics Rapid Release, No. 23*. Hyattsville, MD: National Center for Health Statistics, August 2022.
9 Kochanek KD, Xu J, Arias E. Mortality in the United States, 2019. *Data Brief 395*. Hyattsville, MD: National Center for Health Statistics, 2020.
10 Murphy SL, Kochanek KD, Xu J, Arias E. Mortality in the United States, 2020. *Data Brief 427*. Hyattsville, MD: National Center for Health Statistics, December 2021.
11 Xu J, Murphy SL, Kochanek KD, Arias E. Mortality in the United States, 2021. *Data Brief 456*. Hyattsville, MD: National Center for Health Statistics, December 2022.
12 Hill L, Ndugga V, Artiga S. *Key Data on Health and Health Care by Race and Ethnicity*. San Francisco: Kaiser Family Foundation, March 15, 2023.
13 Woolf SH, Aron L (eds). *National Research Council, Commission on Population. United States Health in International Perspective: Shorter Lives, Poorer Health*. Washington, DC: National Academies Press, 2013.
14 Woolf SH. Necessary but not sufficient: why health care alone cannot improve population health and reduce health inequities. *Ann Fam Med* 2019; 17: 196–199.

15 Smedley BD, Stith AY, Nelson AR (eds). *Unequal Treatment: Confronting Racial and Ethnic Disparities in Health Care.* Washington, DC: National Academies Press, 2003.
16 Ward S, Ngui MM, Bridgewater FD, Harley AE. "You learn to go last": perceptions of prenatal care experiences among African American women with limited incomes. *Matern Child Health J* 2013; 17: 1753–1759.
17 James SA. Confronting the moral economy of US racial/ethnic health disparities. *Am J Public Health* 2003; 93: 189.
18 Geronimus AT. Weathering and age patterns of allostatic load scores among blacks and whites in the United States. *Am J Public Health* 2006; 96: 826–833.
19 Woolf SH. Progress in achieving health equity requires attention to root causes. *Health Aff* 2017; 36: 984–991.
20 Bailey ZD, Feldman JM, Bassett MT. How structural racism works- racist policies as a root cause of US racial health inequities. *NEJM* 2021; 384: 768–773.
21 Barry-Jester AM. The CDC scientist who couldn't get Monkeypox treatment. *ProPublica*, October 5, 2022.
22 *Peristats, Perinatal Data Center, U S Report Card.* Arlington, VA: March of Dimes, 2022.
23 Orr ST, Reiter JP, James SA, Orr CA. Maternal health prior to pregnancy and preterm birth among urban, low-income Black women in Baltimore: the Baltimore Preterm Birth Study. *Ethn Dis* 2011; 22: 85–89.
24 Orr ST, Blackmore-Prince C, James SA, et al. Race, clinical factors, and pregnancy outcomes in a low-income setting. *Ethn Dis* 2000; 10: 411–417.
25 Kim FY, Dagher RK, Chen J. Racial/ ethnic differences in unintended pregnancy: evidence from a national survey of U.S. women. *Am J Prev Med* 2016; 50: 427–435.
26 Orr ST, Miller CA, James SA, Babones S. Unintended pregnancy and preterm birth. *Paediatr Perinat Epidemiol* 2000; 14: 309–313.
27 *Nowhere to Go: Maternity Care Deserts in the United States.* Arlington, VA: March of Dimes (Report), 2022.
28 Starfield B, Shi L. The medical home, access to care, and insurance: a review of evidence. *Pediatrics* 2004; 113 (5 Suppl): 1493–1498.
29 Ho M, Bryson CL, Rumsfeld JS. Medication adherence: its importance in cardiovascular outcomes. *Circulation* 2009; 119: 3028–3035.
30 Carroll L. U.S. heart patients cut back on life-saving drugs due to cost. *Reuters*, 2019.
31 Hall WY, Chapman MV, Lee KM, et al. Implicit racial/ethnic bias among health care professionals and its influence on health care outcomes: a systematic review. *Am J Public Health* 2015; 105: 60–76.
32 Purnell T, Irving W, Irving S, et al. Honoring Dr. Shalom Irving, a champion for health equity. *Health Aff* 2022; 41: 304–308.
33 Cotton TM. I was pregnant and in crisis and all the doctors saw was an incompetent Black woman. *Time*, January 5, 2019.
34 Goelin SK, Yatchmink YE. Maternal depression is a mental health crisis: the time to act is now. *Pediatrics* 2020; 146: e202001413.
35 American College of Obstetrics and Gynecology. Committee opinion number 630: screening for perinatal depression. *Obstet Gynecol* 2015; 125: 1268–1271.
36 United States Preventive Services Task Force. Screening for depression: recommendations and rationale. *Ann Inter Med* 2002; 136: 760–764.

37 United States Preventive Services Task Force. Screening for depression in adults: recommendation statement. *Am Fam Phys* 2016; 94 (4). Published online August 15, 2016.
38 *Biden-Harris Administration Blueprint for Addressing the Maternal Health Crisis*. Washington, DC, 2022.
39 Satcher D, Higgenbotham EJ. The public health approach to eliminating disparities in health. *Am J Public Health* 2008; 98 (Suppl): S8–S11.

11 Conclusions

Introduction

The pandemic of COVID-19, which swept across the United States beginning in the early weeks of 2020, disproportionately burdened Black compared to White women with severe illness and death. The mortality of Black women from COVID-19 was much higher than the mortality among their White counterparts. There are multiple reasons for the disproportionate mortality from COVID-19 among Black compared to White women. Overall, the excess and often preventable deaths among Black compared to White women are caused by the life circumstances and social environment of young Black women. In addition, young Black women are more likely to have other underlying health problems, such as hypertension or diabetes, than their White counterparts. These underlying health conditions among Black women increased the risk of severe illness or death from COVID-19. The pandemic revealed long-standing racial disparities in health in the United States. It also worsened existing disparities in health and further undermined the economic stability of Black families (1).

Much of the focus on improving the health of young Black women has been upon medical care. However, in order to improve the health of young Black women in a meaningful way, there is a need to focus instead on more "upstream" factors and the life conditions that place Black women at increased risk compared to White women of mortality from COVID-19 and other health conditions as well (2). Many of the factors that cause diminished health, decreased life expectancy, and increased mortality among Black compared to White women are found outside of the health care system. These factors are found in the social, economic, physical, and political environment and conditions over the life course of Black women. The deterioration of health among young Black women as they age from their adolescent years into their twenties and thirties, a phenomenon termed "weathering," suggests that exposure to chronic severe social, economic, and environmental stressors year after year takes a growing toll on the health of young Black women, causing premature aging and diminished health (3).

DOI:10.4324/9781032663807-11

An overall belief in the United States has been that harmful health conditions and behaviors (such as obesity, alcohol use, and drug use) are the result of personal weakness and personal decisions. An alternative belief is that exposure to racism and other social stressors over the life course of Black women are the result of current and historical policies and policy decisions, as well as stressful economic and social life conditions.

Social Determinants of Health

Research about Social Determinants of Health has clearly shown that factors in the social, political, economic, and physical environment create conditions that lead to poor health outcomes among young Black women. There is consensus overall in the literature in public health, social epidemiology, and the social sciences that the following factors in the social and physical environment pose risk for harmful health outcomes among young Black women:

- Exposure to racism and other chronic, harmful social stressors (4). Exposure to racism and other social stressors has been shown to increase the risk of depression, preterm birth, and other deleterious physical and mental health outcomes.
- Depression, which occurs more frequently among young Black than young White women, also increases the risk for various serious health conditions, such as cardiovascular disease, cancer, and preterm birth.
- Poverty, economic insecurity, and job insecurity. Black women are more likely to be poor than White women, which increases their risk of unhealthy living conditions and many harmful health conditions. Financial and job insecurity are sources of chronic stressors among young Black women (5).
- Poor educational opportunities. Lack of educational opportunities has negative impacts upon health in several ways. Lack of educational opportunities can create inter-generational poverty. Programs are needed to facilitate early childhood education and child development. Education also improves health literacy for Black women, helping them to live healthier lives.
- Exposure to toxic physical environments by young Black women. Prior research has shown that many young Black women live in neighborhoods that are contaminated with lead in the dust and pollution from automobiles. This exposure to noxious physical agents is more common among young Black than young White women and can have very harmful effects upon health.

Approaches to Reducing Health Inequities Between Young Black and White Women

Several activities and approaches have been suggested as ways to improve the health of young Black women and to reduce inequities in health between young Black and White women. Williams and others have emphasized the importance of focusing upon those "upstream" factors in the social, economic, physical, neighborhood, political, and educational environments that have negative impacts upon health (2). Most of the factors with the greatest impact upon health are found outside the health care system (5–8).

In 1975, at the Annual Meeting of the American Public Health Association, Dr. C. Arden Miller (the President of the American Public Health Association), in his Presidential Address, described a talk given by pediatrician Dr. Jesse Bierman as she was honored by receiving the Martha May Eliot Award in 1968. Dr. Bierman discussed the importance of "upstream" factors outside of the health care system as significant determinants of maternal and child health. She specifically mentioned the harm to health caused by poor-quality housing, population density (overcrowding), and poor-quality education. These three factors are disproportionately faced by Black and low-income families and prevent them from achieving their best health. Dr. Miller urged those who work in maternal and child health and Public Health to focus on these social factors, and on creating "societal change," in order to create an environment in which optimal health can be achieved (9). Achieving health equity will require environments in which all individuals have equal opportunities to obtain their best possible health.

Dr. Bierman and Dr. Miller were ahead of their time in describing these upstream social, economic, and neighborhood factors that harmed health. These factors are now included as Social Determinants of Health. Moreover, for the most part, these social factors cannot be addressed by the health care system in the United States. The United States spends more per capita on health care than other high-income countries yet has poorer health outcomes (such as life expectancy at birth or infant mortality).

Dr. Miller, in his Presidential Address, also recalled that pediatrician Grover Powers, M.D. (in 1949), required residents in Pediatrics at Yale to make a visit to the homes of all newborns discharged after birth at the Yale-New Haven Hospital. Dr. Powers educated the pediatricians he was training that understanding health requires understanding society. His goal was to create healthy people in a healthy society (9). However, as discussed by Dr. Miller, creating a healthy society would require social change to support children and families (9).

Infrastructure and programs to improve the health of young Black women have been woefully underfunded. Changes in upstream programs and expenditures are needed to improve the health of young Black women and reduce health inequities between young Black and White women. These changes include:

- Linking epidemiology, social epidemiology, and public health to the development of policies and programs. This includes measuring and defining racial disparities and inequities in health between young Black and White women.

- Reducing exposure to racism and other chronic, harmful social stressors among young Black women. Exposure to racism and other social stressors has been shown to increase the risk of depression, preterm birth, and other deleterious health outcomes.
- Reducing poverty, economic instability, and income inequality among young Black compared to young White women.
- Providing access to quality child development and education programs for Black children.
- Providing access to affordable, quality, less-crowded housing in safe neighborhoods with reduced crime, violence, and pollution.
- Providing access to stores with fresh, nutritious, healthy foods in the neighborhoods where young Black women live.
- Providing greater regulation of industries that harm health, such as guns (safer policies of sales and storage) and pollution.
- Providing dependable transportation in areas in which young Black women reside.
- Screening for depression among pregnant and postpartum women, and mothers of young children. Depression, which occurs more frequently among young Black than young White women, increases the risk for various serious health conditions, such as cardiovascular disease, cancer, and poor pregnancy outcomes. Pediatricians, obstetrician/gynecologists, and other providers of health care have been urged to screen pregnant and postpartum women and mothers of young children for depression and to refer for treatment when needed (10–13).

There is also a need to develop scientific evidence for the impact of various programs and policies upon the health of Black women (14). Programs should be shown to demonstrate health improvements among young Black women and to reduce health inequities. Policies and programs should give young Black women the best opportunities possible to achieve optimal health (15, 16).

Political Will to Reduce Health Inequities

Woolf has noted that the United States is not lacking in solutions to reduce inequities in health between young Black and White women. Rather, the political will to develop, implement, and evaluate programs and policies to reduce racial inequities is lacking. Woolf continues that Americans need to decide if we are "going to accept being less healthy than other countries" or enact programs and policies to improve health as well as achieve health equity (17).

Prioritizing the Needs of Young Black Women

There has been substantial underinvestment in the health of young Black women. In order to improve the health of young Black women, their needs must be prioritized so that they can achieve the best health possible. Improving the health of young Black women will also result in improved outcomes of their pregnancies, since the health of the mother is a major determinant of the health of a baby.

The Biden White House recently released a "Blueprint for Addressing the Maternal Health Crisis" (18). Among the components of this Blueprint are to:

- Create extended coverage for postpartum care (This will foster a healthier postpartum period and reduce risk of maternal mortality in the postpartum period.);
- Increase investment in maternal health care in rural areas;
- Create additional mental health and substance use treatment resources;
- Improve data on maternal health;
- Increase social services for women.

In order to improve disparate health indicators in the United States, which show the health inequities between young Black and young White women, there is a need for moral and political commitment to create an environment that allows young Black women to achieve health equity (14–17). This is a social justice issue.

The Public Health Approach to Achieving Health Equity

Former Surgeon General David Satcher, M.D., wrote that eliminating health inequities and achieving health equity will require taking a broad public health approach, attacking all determinants of health (15). The public health approach involves:

- Defining and measuring the health problem;
- Determining the causes or risk factors for the problem;
- Determining the best approaches and strategies to ameliorate the problem;
- Implementing and evaluating strategies to improve health.

By using the public health approach described by Miller (9), Satcher and Higgenbotham (15), and others, to address health disparities among young Black women, it will be possible to make progress toward achieving health equity so that the large health inequities between young Black and White women can be eliminated. It will also be possible to create healthy individuals and families in a healthy society (9). Achieving health equity will be a major challenge for the future for the field of Public Health (14, 16). These improvements will save the lives of thousands of Americans who unnecessarily die each year from preventable causes (19–24).

James discussed the public health work needed to reduce racial disparities in health by first undoing racism. He noted that research in public health can provide the evidence to confront and dismantle racism, and thereby eliminate racial inequities in health. James continued, "If, through this work, we provide the American public with sound empirical evidence," that can be used to alter the norms that undergird racism, "It will be one of the finest examples imaginable of science at work in the service of society" (14).

The data presented in this book clearly demonstrate the large and troubling disparities in health between young Black and young White women. These disparities negatively affect their children, families, and communities. The next step in public health research is to create a society without such inequities, with healthy women, pregnancies, infants, and families. Data about the health of other high-resource countries show that it is possible to have a healthier society (21). The United States needs the political will and commitment to no longer accept racial discrimination and health inequities as the norm and to move forward to address and improve the Social Determinants of Health. As noted by Satcher and Higgenbotham, "We all have a role to play" (15). The steps we take and policy changes we implement will save and improve lives of young Black women and lead to health equity, social change, and social justice.

References

1 Frye J. *On the Frontlines at Work and at Home: The Disproportionate Effects of the Coronavirus Pandemic on Women of Color*. Washington, DC: Center for American Progress, April 23, 2020.
2 Williams DR, Costa MV, Odunlami AO, Mohammed SA. Moving upstream: how interventions that address the social determinants of health can improve health and racial disparities. *J Public Health Manag Pract*. 2008; 14 (Suppl): S8–S17.
3 Geronimus AT. Understanding and eliminating racial inequalities in women's health in the United States: the role of the weathering conceptual framework. *J Am Med Womens Assoc* 2001; 56: 133–136.
4 Orr ST, James SA, Casper R. Psychosocial stressors and low birthweight: development of a questionnaire. *J Dev Behav Pediatr* 1992; 13: 343–347.
5 American Public Health Association. Structural racism is a public health crisis: impact on the Black community. *APHA Policy Statement Number LB20–04*, October 24, 2020.
6 Williams DR, Lawrence JA, Davis BA. Racism and health: evidence and needed research. *Annu Rev Public Health* 2019; 40: 105–125.
7 Bailey ZD, Krieger N, Agenor M, et al. Structural racism and health inequities in the USA: evidence and interventions. *Lancet* 2017; 389: 1453–1463.
8 Williams DR, Lawrence JA, Davis BA, Vu C. Understanding how discrimination can affect health. *Health Serv Res* 2019; 54: 1374–1388.
9 Miller CA. Societal change and public health: a rediscovery. *Am J Public Health* 1976; 66: 54–60.
10 Goelein SK, Yatchmink YE. Maternal depression is a mental health crisis: the time to act is now. *Pediatrics* 2020; 146: e202001413.

11 American College of Obstetrics and Gynecology Committee Opinion Number 630. Screening for perinatal depression. *Obstetr Gynecol* 2015; 125: 1268–1271.
12 United States Preventive Services Task Force. Screening for depression: recommendations and rationale. *Ann Intern Med* 2002; 136: 760–764.
13 United States Preventive Services Task Force. Screening for depression in adults: recommendation statement. *Am Fam Phys* 2016; 94. Published online August 15, 2016.
14 James SA. Confronting the moral economy of US racial/ethnic health disparities. *Am J Public Health* 2003; 93: 185–187.
15 Satcher D, Higginbotham EJ. The public health approach to eliminating disparities in health. *Am J Public Health* 2008; 98 (Suppl): S8–S11.
16 Williams DR, Purdie-Vaughns V. Needed interventions to reduce racial/ethnic disparities in health. *J Health Polit Policy Law* 2016; 41: 627–651.
17 Weintraub K. Americans' life expectancy continues to fall, erasing health gains of the last quarter century. *USA Today*, December 22, 2022.
18 *Biden White House Blueprint for Addressing the Maternal Health Crisis*, June 2022.
19 Braveman PA, Arkin E, Proctor D, et al. Systemic and structural racism: definitions, examples, health damages, and approaches to dismantling. *Health Aff* 2022; 41: 171–178.
20 Chinn JJ, Martin IK, Redmond N. Health equity among Black women in the United States. *J Womens Health* 2021; 30: 212–219.
21 Woolf SH, Aron L (eds). *National Research Council, Commission on Population. United States Health in International Perspective: Shorter Lives, Poorer Health.* Washington, DC: National Academies Press, 2013.
22 Woolf SH. Falling behind: the growing gap in life expectancy between the United States and other countries, 1933–2021. *Am J Public Health* 2023; e1–e11.
23 Galea S, Tracy M, Hoggert KJ. Estimated deaths attributable to social factors in the United States. *Am J Public Health* 2011; 101: 1456–1465.
24 Woolf SH. Excess deaths will continue until the root causes are addressed. *Health Aff* 2022; 41: 1562–1564.

Index

Note: Page numbers in **bold** indicate tables.

MIX

Papier | Fördert gute Waldnutzung

FSC® C083411

Kolibri 360 GmbH
Ferdinand-Jühlke-Straße 7
99095 Erfurt, Deutschland
produktsicherheit@kolibri360.de